Risk, communication and health psychology

Health psychology

Series editors:
Sheila Payne and Sandra Horn

Published titles

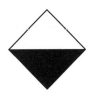

Risk, communication and health psychology

Dianne C. Berry

Open University Press

Open University Press
McGraw-Hill Education
McGraw-Hill House
Shoppenhangers Road
Maidenhead
Berkshire
SL6 2QL

email: enquiries@openup.co.uk
world wide web: www.openup.co.uk

and Two Penn Plaza, New York, NY 10121-2289, USA

First Published 2004

A catalogue record of this book is available from the British Library

ISBN 0 335 21315 0 (pb)   0 335 21352 9 (hb)

Library of Congress Cataloging-in-Publication Data
CIP data has been applied for

Typeset by RefineCatch Ltd, Bungay, Suffolk
Printed in the UK by Bell & Bain Ltd, Glasgow

Joyce Willock

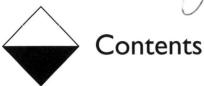

Contents

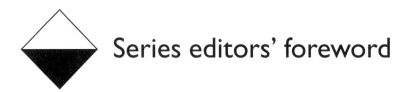

Series editors' foreword

This series of books in health psychology is designed to support post-graduate and postqualification studies in psychology, nursing, medicine and paramedical sciences as well as health psychology units in the undergraduate curriculum. Health psychology has grown, and continues to grow, rapidly as a field of study. Concerned as it is with the application of psychological theories and models to the promotion and maintenance of health, and the individual and interpersonal aspects of adaptive behaviour in illness and disability, health psychology has a wide remit and a potentially important role to play in the future.

Risk and risk behaviour are central issues in maintaining positive health and managing ill health, but there is a dearth of good relevant books on the topic. The perception, communication and management of risks to health provide a number of challenges, not least of which is presenting the concept of risk so that it can be understood readily. This book is a timely and welcome addition to the series. It is written in an accessible style and is designed to appeal to a wide audience. A special feature of the book is that it brings together a range of material previously covered in separate texts.

Professor Dianne Berry has drawn on her own extensive research and that of others to produce an up-to-date and evidence-based text, which is also engaging and enjoyable to read. She begins by considering the dilemmas inherent in patient empowerment and shared decision making, and goes on to consider different perspectives on, and models of, risk. The next chapters cover influencing health behaviours, communicating information about health and treatment, and communicating probabilistic information – a core topic and one which has challenged generations of health educators. Professor Berry then discusses the use of patient information leaflets and other ways of conveying and assessing risk. The book ends by drawing together information on 'where we are now' with regard to risk, and out-lines future challenges and opportunities.

Better information about how risk is conveyed, understood and translated into health behaviours is a key function of health psychology. For this reason, we welcome this book as an exciting addition to the series.

Sheila Payne and Sandra Horn

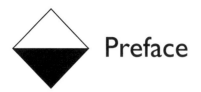 # Preface

I had planned to start writing this book in the summer of 2003 but, in my enthusiasm for the project, I started the preceding Christmas and had virtually finished it by the summer. I was helped by being a naturally early riser, as most of the hours were put in before the rest of my family were awake each day. At the start of this preface, I should make it clear why I am so interested in risk communication in relation to health. In my view, risk touches on virtually every aspect of our health and lives, and the need for effective communication is paramount. I very much hope that if you have not appreciated this already, by the end of this book, you will.

I first became interested in risk and health communication, particularly in relation to medicine taking, in the mid- to late 1990s. I had been invited to take part in an EC-funded research project which involved developing an intelligent computer system for drug prescription. My group's role in the project was to advise on the content of, and to evaluate, the written explanations that would be generated by the system. We started with two simple questions: what do people want to know about their medicines, and what should they be told? As experimental psychologists we naturally took a very empirical approach to answering the questions and, from the first experiment on, I was hooked. This book attempts to answer these questions, as well as a number of broader questions relating to the communication of risk information in health.

I decided to write this book as a result of my general dissatisfaction with most existing texts in the area. Although several contained one or two chapters of interest, none seemed to cover the particular issues that interested me most, in a single volume. I therefore set out to do this, and the present book is the result. I hope that it will be of interest to fellow researchers, practitioners and students, who want to know more about the communication of risk information in health.

This book draws on material from several different disciplines, including psychology, sociology, health, medicine, pharmacy, statistics, and business and management. After making the case for why risk communication is so important in relation to health, it looks in more detail at what we mean by risk and at the different theories that have been put forward to explain it. The book also considers the different methods for communicating risk and the influence of these on people's health behaviours, particularly medicine taking. It covers communication between individuals as well as risk communication at the broader public health level. Although the focus of the book is on risk communication, it naturally touches on the related areas of risk assessment and risk management and, in the final chapter, looks at many of the interesting ethical issues that are raised by this important topic.

Although this is a single-authored text, a number of others have contributed to my thinking in this area. First, a long-standing colleague and now dear friend, Fiorella de Rosis from the University of Bari in Italy invited me to join the EC project on developing the drug prescription system. She and her colleagues worked with my group in Oxford and then Reading in developing and evaluating the explanations. Tony Gillie, Irene Michas and Jeanette Garwood worked closely with me on this project, and each played an important role. Following this, Irene Michas and I received funding from the UK's Medical Research Council to take the work further. The particular focus of the project was investigating the effects of providing people with different information, in different forms, about medication side-effects. Elisabetta Bersellini, who has continued to work with me for the past five years, was employed as the research fellow. I am very grateful to Beba (as she is known) for all that she has contributed over this time. More recently, I have also worked with several other research assistants and Ph.D. students in Reading – Hedwig Natter, Natalie Lynch, Elizabeth Dixon and Paula Brown, and some of their work is referred to in the chapters that follow.

One research collaboration that has been particularly productive over the past three years stemmed from an invitation to speak at a symposium, organized by Lynn Myers, at the British Psychological Society Division of Health Psychology conference in Leeds in the late 1990s. A fellow speaker in the symposium was Theo Raynor, a researcher in the Pharmacy Practice and Medicines Management Group at the University of Leeds. I am exceedingly grateful to Theo, and to his associate Peter Knapp, for what is probably the most productive and enjoyable research collaboration I have had. They have both contributed enormously to my thinking in this area and have motivated me to keep researching and writing on this topic.

When writing a preface, one always tends to leave the most personal thanks to last. I am following this tradition but, as is often the case, last in no way implies least. I am particularly grateful to my husband, John Harris, and to my children, Marc and Kate Berry, for putting up with my early morning starts, when I occasionally disturbed them, and for not complaining about the many heaps of journal articles that constantly littered our house for around six months or so. However, I am especially grateful for their enthusiasm and encouragement. Finally, I am very grateful to my parents, Jean and Maurice Broadfield, for their continuing help and support. Without this, I would never have been able to establish my career while raising a young family, and would not have been in the position, some years later, to write this book.

CHAPTER 1

An introduction to risk communication in health

In 1995 the Committee on Safety of Medicines (CSM) issued a warning that third generation oral contraceptives were associated with 'around twice the risk' compared with second generation preparations. This relatively simple and straightforward risk communication had unexpected and far-reaching effects. In particular, it led to considerable anxiety in many women, and resulted in a dramatic decrease in use of the pill and a steep rise in pregnancies and terminations. The situation was greatly exacerbated by intensive (and unbalanced) media coverage. What was not explained to women at the time was that the absolute level of risk was actually very low, and that the risk of thrombosis in pregnancy was several times higher.

The 'pill scare', as it has become known, clearly illustrates how failure to interpret risk information in the way intended by advisory bodies can have significant and unanticipated detrimental effects on health behaviour. The UK Chief Medical Officer, in his 1996 report, said that a key issue highlighted by the scare was the importance of the distinction between absolute and relative risk (see Chapter 3). However, as Adams (1998: 150) pointed out, 'the more important lesson is that scientists, by combining uncertainty with dire consequences, can frighten large numbers of people'. This is particularly the case when such matters attract media attention and become subject to sensationalized and unbalanced reporting.

Many of the issues touched on above are reflected in subsequent chapters in the present book. We will see how risk communication can have significant effects on health behaviours, and how the particular way in which the information is presented can influence those behaviours. We will also look at how emotions interact with cognitive processes when interpreting health messages. Finally, we will consider the potentially far-reaching effects that communications can have in the present day (particularly with the 'aid' of new technology and media reporting), as well as some of the wider ethical concerns that arise in relation to risk and health communication.

The 'explosion' of interest in risk and in health communication

Over the past 20 years or so, people have become increasingly exposed to information about health, both at an individual and society (public) health level. This can be seen not only in the considerable increase in the number of specialist academic journal articles and books that are being published, but also in terms of the growing availability of information leaflets that accompany medicines or are written about particular medical conditions and treatments. It is also evidenced by the vast number of popular books and magazines devoted to health topics, the increase in specialist television programmes (including a dedicated Sky TV channel in the UK) and the thousands of sites and dedicated pages on the internet. Health communication has also become a core topic in training in nearly all medicine and health related professions. The public, at present, seems to have an insatiable thirst for this flood of information, as evidenced by sales figures of popular books and magazines, TV viewing figures and internet hit rates, as well the large number of empirical studies which have shown that patients want to receive more information about their illnesses and treatments than they are currently given.

During the same period, we have also seen an explosion of interest in the topic of risk, again with increasingly vast amounts being written about the subject. Risk, in some form or another, now features in a high proportion of articles in newspapers, magazines and on TV programmes. Similarly, as we will see in Chapter 2, there has been a sharp increase in the number of academic articles and books devoted to the subject. Businesses have been set up to assess risks and to advise on their management, giving rise to the new profession of 'risk consultant'.

The present book brings these two areas together to focus on risk communication in health. Indeed, much of the current attention to risk concerns health matters. As Calman (2001: 47) recently noted, 'scarcely a day goes past without some scare, risk or alert on a matter of health or health care being raised in the media'. I will shortly explain why risk communication is such an important topic in relation to health but, before this, I will briefly outline what I mean by 'risk'.

What do we mean by 'risk'?

Numerous definitions of risk have been proposed over the past 20 years or so. Some are longer or more complex than others, but the majority feature two main elements: a probabilistic aspect and a negative/hazardous aspect. We will see in Chapter 2 how risk has not always been conceived of in this way, and we will look at how conceptions have changed over time, as well as at the different emphases that currently exist in different disciplines or traditions. For now, I will use one of the most simple definitions that has been advocated, which is the one proposed by the British Medical Association in 1990, namely that 'risk is the probability that something unpleasant will happen' (p.14). Thus, it is not certain that the event will occur (the probabilistic aspect) but, if it does occur, the event will have negative rather than positive consequences (the hazardous aspect).

The present book focuses on risk communication, but clearly there is more to risk than simply communicating information about it. First, risks need to be assessed or measured in some way; these aspects are the focus of the area known as 'risk assessment'. However, people will not necessarily perceive risks in line with these 'objective' assessments/measures; rather, their perceptions are likely to be influenced by a number of subjective elements. Thus, there is also interest in the area known as 'risk perception'. Finally, risks need to be managed by individuals and, particularly, by organizations and institutions, and these aspects are the concern of the area known as 'risk management'. Clearly, these three areas are not distinct from each other, nor from the area of risk communication. In Chapter 2, I will say more about each of these three areas and show how they relate to risk communication.

We can think about risk assessment, perception, management and communication in relation to health, but risk features in many other areas of our lives. For example, we face risks from the environment (e.g. in terms of pollution, energy shortages or natural disasters), from our lifestyles (e.g. in terms of the way we drive, or our sporting activities or diets), and from a host of other interpersonal factors (such as family and sexual relationships). In addition, we are subject to economic and criminal risks, as well as the growing risks arising from new technology. Many of the points that I make in relation to health throughout this book will apply to these other areas as well. In addition, risks that arise in many of these other areas can also impinge on our health and well-being. Indeed, we live in a complex technological world and virtually everything that we do, or is done to us, carries some risk to our health and welfare (British Medical Association 1990).

So why is risk communication so important in relation to health?

According to McGinnis and Foege (1993), of the 2,148,000 deaths that occurred in the USA in 1990, over 40 per cent were due to modifiable factors, such as lifestyle factors (e.g. smoking, poor diet, sedentary lifestyle, excess alcohol, sexual risk behaviour, illicit drug use and motor vehicle accidents). In addition, another 10 per cent were due to modifiable causes such as occupational hazards, environmental pollutants, food contaminants and preventable infectious diseases. Clearly, effective risk communication, at both the individual and public level, can play a key role in relation to reducing the negative influence of these factors. However, the emphasis must be on the word 'effective' because, as the 1995 'pill scare' showed us, risk communications that are inadequate in some way can have significant and unforeseen detrimental effects on people's health behaviours.

Until relatively recently the dominant tradition in doctor–patient communications was what is now commonly referred to as 'paternalism'. According to this model of communication, doctors made all the decisions in relation to a patient's health and treatments and barely even communicated or justified these to patients, let alone involved them in the decision making. In this context, Calman *et al.* (1999: 109) noted that it is a 'poignant footnote to the founding of the NHS [National Health Service] that Nye Bevan should have died of cancer without ever having been told of his diagnosis'.

The move from this 'paternalistic' tradition in health to the current emphasis on patient empowerment and shared decision making has meant that patients want and need reliable, comprehensive and understandable information about their conditions and treatments. This must include information about the risks and benefits of the different treatment options, if patients are to participate fully in decisions about, and share responsibility for, their own health care. Enabling people to make such informed decisions is a cornerstone of the philosophy of concordance in medicine taking and is a key element in the current UK National Plan for the NHS (Department of Health 2000). This plan builds on the earlier *Patient's Charter*, which proposed that patients have a right 'to be given a clear explanation of any treatment proposed, including any risks and any alternatives, before you decide whether you will agree to the treatment' (Department of Health 1992).

Linked to this latter approach is the notion of informed consent. Patients not only have to give consent for particular treatments to be carried out, but there is now clear guidance about the information that they must be given before making their decision. In particular, patients must be given information about:

♦ their diagnosis and likely prognosis if left untreated (including any uncertainties);
♦ options for further investigation;
♦ options for treatment/management (including the option not to treat).

In this latter case they must also be given information about the probability of success or failure of the different options, as well as the different lifestyle changes that might be entailed. Clearly, information about risks and benefits is a key element of this. However, seeking informed consent entails more than simply providing people with the specified information. To make an informed decision, people must be able to understand the information that they are given and apply it to their own circumstances. This holds whether we are considering medicine taking, being vaccinated, undergoing genetic screening and other health tests, as well as the full range of medical and surgical interventions.

The challenge of risk communication

As we will see in subsequent chapters in this book, however, this move towards patient empowerment and informed consent can present doctors and other health professionals with a considerable challenge. This is because many people are not cognitively and/or emotionally equipped to understand, retain and use the necessary information (Doyal 2001). Effectively communicating even the simplest and most unthreatening of messages to a diverse audience is difficult enough, but the problems of communicating complex medical information, involving risk and uncertainty, are immense.

We will see in Chapter 3 how different cognitive limitations and emotional biases can affect the way in which risk information is interpreted. For example, numerous studies have shown that many people (and not just lay people) have difficulty understanding numerical information, particularly when presented as percentages. To give a brief illustration here, consider the following: 'If there is a 50% chance that it will rain on Saturday and a 50% chance that it will rain on Sunday, what is the likelihood that it will rain this weekend?' (Gigerenzer 2002: 23). Gigerenzer described how an American TV weather forecaster mistakenly informed viewers that the chance of rain that weekend was 100 per cent. He also gave the example of a recent German study in which people were asked:

What does 40% mean?
− 1 in 4
− 4 out of every 10
− every 40th person

(Gigerenzer 2002: 23.)

Over a third of the sample of 1000 Germans tested did not select the correct answer. As the UK Secretary of State for Trade and Industry has stated, 'fifty per cent of the public doesn't actually know what 50% means' (the *Independent*, 30 November 2002).

We will see more fully in Chapter 3 that, in addition to these general problems with interpreting probabilistic information, there is also evidence to show that people are subject to a number of specific biases when making their judgements. For example, we are very prone to overestimate the probability of events that are more readily available in memory. For instance, having recently witnessed a road accident, or seen an overturned car at the side of the road, we judge the probability of our being involved in an accident to be much higher. We will also see in Chapter 3 how the particular way in which information is presented can affect people's understanding and decisions. In relation to the 1995 'pill scare', for example, the dramatic effects may not have occurred if women had been told that the increase in risk was from 15 per 100,000 users to 25 per 100,000 users, rather than being told that the risk associated with third generation pills was around twice the level of that associated with earlier preparations.

As a result of difficulties such as these, several researchers and practitioners have recommended particular ways of improving the communication of risk information. Some have tried to establish best practice in relation to the use of more traditional ways of presenting probabilistic information, whereas others have advocated the use of specially devised scales and presentation methods. In addition, as we will see in Chapter 7, many people working in this area are now turning to the use of new technology as a tool for aiding communication and decision making, and particularly for reaching large and diverse audiences. Unfortunately, as will become clear in the later chapters of this book, not all of the recommended advances have been found to lead to the expected improvements in communication, and some have raised other issues – for example, in relation to ethical matters. The challenge for the future will be to develop and implement effective methods that bring about the intended positive effects, while avoiding or minimizing unnecessary and unanticipated negative effects.

Preview of remaining chapters

The remainder of this book expands upon the issues raised in the preceding sections. Chapter 2 looks in more detail at what we mean by risk and at the differences in emphasis in interpretation of the term in different disciplines. It also considers how general usage of the concept has changed over time. The chapter reviews the main theoretical approaches in the area, namely the cognitive science or psychometric perspective, Douglas' sociocultural perspective, the risk society approach associated with the writings of Beck and Giddens and Foucault's governmentality approach. Finally, the chapter briefly looks at the related fields of risk assessment, risk perception and risk management, and at how these relate to the area of risk communication.

Chapter 3 focuses on the question of how to communicate information about risk and considers many of the limitations of existing presentation methods and formats. It starts off by discussing some of the basic cognitive limitations and biases that we are all prone to when interpreting probabilistic information. It then looks at how interpretations are affected by the particular way in which information is presented; for instance, as percentages as opposed to frequencies, using verbal terms as opposed to numbers, as being positively as opposed to negatively framed, and as relative as opposed to absolute values. It also considers the problems experienced when interpreting information about cumulative risk and when attempting to trade off information about risks and benefits. Finally it considers the effects of emotional factors (such as affect and anxiety) on risk judgements, as well as evidence that people are unrealistically optimistic when assessing their own level of risk.

Chapter 4 is concerned with why and how health messages can influence people's health behaviours. It begins by considering some of the main determinants of health and of the outcomes of health care services, and looks at what affects people's perceptions of health. It then reviews the main social cognitive models of health behaviour (namely, the health belief model, theory of planned behaviour, protection motivation theory, the stages of change model and the self-regulatory model), and assesses evidence for the link between perceived risk and behaviour. It looks in particular at the issue of adherence to prescribed medication, given that this is a health behaviour that is engaged in by the vast majority of the population at some time in their lives.

In Chapter 5 we look in more detail at the effects of providing health information. The chapter begins by looking at different styles of doctor–patient communication, before addressing the question of what information people want (and need) to be given about their illnesses and potential treatments. It looks at the effects of providing information on people's knowledge and memory, as well as on their behaviours, including adherence. The chapter then takes medicine as a specific example and looks particularly at the communication of information about medication side-effects. In addition to prescribed medicines, it also considers particular issues that arise in relation to 'over the counter', herbal and homeopathic medicines. Finally, it considers the problems of providing health information to the general public in order to promote better health.

Chapter 6 expands on the topic of patient information and looks in detail at written information and, particularly, at patient information leaflets and at the main issues relating to their comprehension and use. It reviews a number of studies that have evaluated the quality and availability of such materials and summarizes key design considerations and existing guidelines in relation to good practice. It looks in particular at the communication of risk information in medicine information leaflets. It provides an overview of the regulations and recommendations that have been produced in different countries across the world (e.g. the European Union (EU) America, Australia) in relation to the development and distribution of such leaflets. It focuses on the recent European Commission guidelines, which make recommendations in relation to the content and format of medicine information leaflets, and describes a set of empirical studies that have been carried out to evaluate their main recommendations. Finally, it considers some principles and wider implications that can be drawn from these studies.

Chapter 7 reviews a number of other risk scales and methods for conveying risk information, in addition to the numerical and verbal methods outlined in the preceding chapter, including risk ladders, Calman and Royston's Community scale and Barclay et al.'s Lottery scale. It also looks at a number of more traditional graphical presentation methods and assesses their relative merits. The chapter then considers the more general use of computers to aid the interpretation of risk and health information, including the recent development of a number of computerized decision aids. Finally, it addresses some of the wider implications of using new technology, including the internet, to communicate health and risk information.

The final chapter starts by returning to the 1995 'pill scare' and assesses why it happened and what can be done to prevent similar events occurring in the future. In doing this, it brings together many of the key points that have been highlighted in the preceding chapters, such as the role of emotional as well as cognitive limitations, the importance of personal values and the issue of trust in risk communicators. It then looks at what can and should be done to improve communication. As might be expected, much of the discussion involves setting out future challenges rather than offering ready-made solutions. Finally, it considers a number of ethical issues that arise in relation to communicating risk information in health.

Defining and explaining risk

CHAPTER
2

In Chapter 1 we described risk as 'the probability that something unpleasant will happen' (following the definition put forward by the British Medical Association in 1990). In this chapter we expand on this definition and on the different uses of the term, and show how its meaning has changed over time. We also look at different theoretical models of risk, as well as at issues that arise in the assessment, perception and management of risk, and how these relate to the problem of how to communicate information about risk effectively.

Definition and usage of the term 'risk'

One of the most frequently quoted definitions of risk, particularly in relation to health and safety, is that set down by the Royal Society Study Group in 1983. They defined risk as the 'probability that a particular adverse event occurs during a stated period of time, or results from a particular challenge. As a probability in the sense of statistical theory, risk obeys all the formal laws of combining probabilities' (Adams 1995: 8). The Study Group distinguished between the risk itself and the 'harm' experienced as a result of an adverse event. In doing so, they defined 'detriment' as 'a numerical measure of the expected harm or loss associated with an adverse event . . . It is generally the integrated product of risk and harm and is often expressed in terms such as costs in pounds, loss in expected years of life or loss of productivity, and is needed for numerical exercises such as cost-benefit analysis or risk-benefit analysis' (Adams 1995: 8). Thus, these are very 'objective' definitions that allow little room for the role of subjective perceptions and experiences. We will see shortly that not everyone interprets and uses the term 'risk' in this way.

Usage of the term 'risk' varies, or is at least given different types of emphasis in different scientific disciplines. In epidemiology, for example, the main emphasis in relation to risk is on identifying and measuring the negative consequences of events, whereas in statistics the emphasis is primarily on measuring and predicting the probability or chance of specific events occurring. Similarly, engineering tends to be concerned with the relationship between positive and negative consequences of events and often involves balancing potential benefits with risks in order to establish tolerable levels of risk. Finally, in social science the emphasis is typically on studying the ways that individuals and groups identify and respond to risk. As can be seen, some disciplines are very much concerned with objective measurable aspects whereas others (primarily social scientists) also allow for consideration of more subjective aspects.

Changing conceptions of risk over time

The term 'risk' has not always been used in the above way or ways. The main sources of risk and ways of controlling it have changed over the centuries. In the Middle Ages, the major perceived risks were associated with natural events and acts of God, such as floods and epidemics. During the eighteenth and nineteenth centuries, the concept became increasingly scientific and was also extended to cover man–made events and human activities and relationships. People started to try to measure and predict risks. During this period, the term was also used to describe potentially positive events (such as investments) as well negative ones. However, the second half of the twentieth century saw a narrowing in the use of the term so that it is now virtually always used in association with negative or dangerous events (as was apparent in the definitions given earlier).

The pervasiveness of risk

As noted in Chapter 1, over the past 20 to 30 years our attention has been increasingly drawn to the diverse range of risks that we face in our everyday lives. The amount of information that is communicated in writing, or via TV and other media, has been growing almost exponentially. Much of this is in the area of human health. In terms of scientific articles, Skolbekken (1995: 297) has referred to 'the risk epidemic in medical journals' (see also Edwards et al. 1998a). He reports a search of MEDLINE databases which shows a dramatic increase in the number of publications with the term 'risk' in the title or abstract between 1967 and 1991. There is no sign that this 'epidemic' has levelled off over the past decade. Lupton (1999) noted a marked increase in use of the term 'risk' in the main text and headlines of articles published in Australian newspapers between 1992 and 1997. Similarly, Adams (1995) described how UK newspapers and TV programmes are dominated by items that refer to risk. A skim through current newspapers and TV programmes will show that the situation is still continuing (at least in the westernized world).

Nearly all of our activities carry some level of risk, from our earliest years. A young infant learning to crawl or take the first few steps, or a young child learning to swim or ride a bicycle or a horse can be viewed as a serious risk management exercise. Throughout childhood, there is usually a gradual handing over of responsibility for risk from parents to their off-spring. Children learn to cross roads, travel alone and determine which activities they should engage in and which they should avoid. During this process, they learn to find the right balance between risk and reward. As many 'risky' activities will also have potentially negative consequences for people other than the individual concerned, in most societies there is also a third tier of responsibility for risk. Thus, there are a number of authorities and regulatory bodies that institute policies, regulations and laws (e.g. in relation to anti-pollution, compulsory wearing of seatbelts and drinking and driving) that influence many aspects of our environments and lives.

Basic dimensions of risk

Bogardus *et al.* (1999) identified five different fundamental dimensions of risk as follows:

Identity

Some risks are known (e.g. the probability of developing a thromboembo-lism if you take the oral contraceptive pill), whereas others (particularly where new therapies and technologies are concerned) may not be known. Empirical studies have shown that people are particularly concerned about unknown risks (e.g. Slovic 1987; Bennett 1998).

Permanence

Some risks have permanent effects (such as death) while other effects are only temporary (e.g. developing an infection following an operation, or feeling nauseous while taking a particular medicine).

Timing

Unwarranted effects may occur immediately, or after several weeks, months, or even years, as in the case of new variant Creutzfeldt–Jakob disease (CJD), the human form of bovine spongiform encephalopathy (BSE).

Probability

Risks differ in terms of the likelihood with which they occur. We will see in Chapter 3 that these likelihoods can be expressed in various different ways (e.g. numerically, verbally, graphically), with the different formats influencing people's interpretations.

Value

Different people attach different values to particular risks. What one person judges to be catastrophic may be viewed as a necessary inconvenience by another. These subjective values affect how people interpret and respond to different risks. Linked to this is the extent to which risks are thought to be justifiable as opposed to unjustifiable (see e.g. Calman 1996).

In addition to these five dimensions, risks also differ in the extent to which they are avoidable. For example, it is relatively easy to avoid taking a recreational drug or engaging in unprotected sex, but it is less easy to avoid being at risk of an earthquake if you live in San Francisco. Risks also differ in the extent to which they have indirect as well as direct consequences (as portrayed in Kasperson *et al.*'s 1988 social amplification model, which will be discussed later in this chapter).

Calman (1996) proposed that risks also differ in the extent to which they are serious as opposed to non-serious, in that some can have life-threatening consequences whereas others would be considered to be relatively minor. Clearly, at the margin, assessing seriousness is likely to involve a subjective as well as objective judgement. As we will see in Chapter 6, Calman proposed a Verbal Risk scale, ranging from '*negligible*' to '*high*', where '*negligible*' is used to describe an adverse event occurring in less that one per million episodes or treatments and '*high*' to describe a risk of greater than one in a hundred (see Table 2.1). Calman pointed out that, although *negligible* risks may be considered to be remote or insignificant, one should never use the word 'safe' in this context. Similarly, the British Medical Association (1990) noted that everything that we do, or is done to us, carries some risk to our health and welfare: 'There is no such thing as zero risk or absolutely safety' (p. xiv).

Our perception of risk, and the way we react to it, are likely to depend on a range of factors including our previous experiences and values, and the

Table 2.1 Calman's (1996) proposed Verbal Risk scale

Frequency label	Designated band (%)
High	> 1
Moderate	0.1–1
Low	0.01–0.1
Very Low	0.001–0.01
Minimal	0.0001–0.001
Negligible	< 0.0001

culture in which we live. At no time will all of us agree on a single level of acceptable risk. What is viewed as a risk by one individual or society may not be viewed in the same way by another. Lupton (1999), for example, described how many heroin addicts are aware of the risks associated with the drug itself, but see the repeated injections (often using unclean needles) as routine, virtually risk-free, daily events. As outlined below, the notion that risk perception and interpretation are affected, to some extent, by people's values and are a function of the social and historical context is a key element in some, although not all, of the leading theoretical accounts of risk.

Risk theories

Risk theories can be grouped into two main classes: the technico-scientific/ cognitive science approach and the sociocultural perspective. The main difference between them concerns the extent to which risk probabilities are treated as objective facts, as opposed to being constructed within a particular social and cultural perspective.

Cognitive science approach

According to this approach, risks (typically hazards) exist in the world and can be identified through scientific measurement and calculation. They can also be managed or controlled using this knowledge. Calculations of probability are a major element of the approach, with there being very little, if any, allowance for any subjective element. Thus, the risk or hazard is seen as the 'objective' variable, and an individual's reaction to it as the 'subjective' variable. Particular people and bodies (e.g. medical doctors, financial analysts, the Food Standards Agency) are assumed, because of their previous training and experience, to be risk experts whose knowledge about risk is based on scientific understanding, and is therefore 'valued'. In contrast, lay people tend to be portrayed as responding unscientifically to risk and as being in need of education in relation to particular risks and ways of controlling them, particularly when their perceptions of risk differ from those of the 'experts'. As Sjoberg (1997: 128) argued, models such as these tend to paint a picture of the public as 'emotional, arbitrary and irrational', and their perceptions of risk as subjective and frequently inaccurate and invalid.

In general, the cognitive science perspective uses psychological models of human behaviour to understand how people interpret and react to par-ticular risks. Within this approach, the psychometric perspective identifies various mental strategies, or heuristics, that people use when perceiving and interpreting risks. The health belief model (e.g. Rosenstock 1966, 1974) and protection motivation theory (e.g. Rogers 1975), for example, can be considered to be 'psychometric risk models' in that they primarily represent human behaviour as being rational and volitional (see Chapter 4 for more detail). According to these models, there is a linear relationship between factors such as a person's perceptions about the severity of a risk and their acknowledgement that they are personally at risk, and their decision to adopt a behaviour to reduce or prevent the risk.

Another feature of the cognitive science approach is that it tends to focus very much at the level of the individual person. Perceptions depend on how individuals view and understand the world and do not take account of the ways in which cultural conceptual categories mediate their interpretation. People perceive and respond to risks as individuals rather than as members of a particular group, organization or culture. Similarly, risks themselves tend to be viewed as individual entities, separate from other risks and behaviours.

Sociocultural perspectives

Although the dominant scientific view (often held by physical scientists) is that risks can be objectively defined and measured, other writers (particularly social scientists) have argued that risk is culturally constructed, in that both the adverse nature of particular events and their probability of occurrence are inherently subjective. Not everyone will perceive a risk in the same way. Thus, sociocultural perspectives emphasize the social and cultural context within which risks are perceived, understood and controlled. Lupton (1999) distinguished between three major classes of sociocultural theory, namely the cultural symbolic perspective (e.g. Douglas 1992), the risk society perspective (e.g. Giddens 1990, 1991; Beck 1992) and the governmentality perspective (e.g. Foucault 1991). As Lupton pointed out, common to all three perspectives is the notion that risk has become an increasingly pervasive concept of human existence in western societies and is seen as a central cultural and political concept by which individuals, social groups and institutions are organized and regulated.

The cultural symbolic perspective

In essence, this approach emphasizes that risk judgements are political, moral and aesthetic, and are constructed through frameworks of understanding. It goes beyond the individual to adopt a shared social and cultural approach. The key exponent, Mary Douglas, has argued that perception of, and responses to, risk are related to an individual's position in a cultural system (e.g. Douglas 1992). There are no fixed objective measures of risk, as each individual and each society will define and perceive risk in a different way. According to Douglas, differences in risk interpretation between experts and lay people should not be attributed to the lay people's cognitive limitations or lack of knowledge or understanding, but to the fact that other (frequently valid) concerns are brought to bear on, and influence, their judgements. Much of Douglas' writings have focused on why some hazards are perceived as risks by certain people whereas others are not, and she draws on a range of social and cultural factors to explain this. In general, her approach has been very influential, although it has been criticized for being too static and for not accounting sufficiently for change (e.g. Lupton 1999).

Sjoberg (1997) reviewed evidence for the cultural theory of risk perception by comparing risk judgements in two different cultures (Sweden and Brazil). Contrary to expectations based on cultural theory, it was found that perceived risk was a function of 'real life' rather than being determined by culturally contingent values and beliefs. He concluded that cultural theory explains only a very minor share of the variance of perceived risk and that it adds even less to what is explained by different approaches.

The risk society perspective

A second sociocultural approach is referred to as the risk society perspective. This approach focuses on processes such as individualization, reflexivity and globalization. It considers the politics and macro level of the current meanings and strategies of risk. Risk is seen as a central concern in the modern era, emerging from the processes of modernization. In such a society, people tend to be more concerned with preventing 'bad' things that might occur than with bringing about good things. The writings of the two leading theorists associated with this approach (Ulrich Beck and Anthony Giddens) have much in common, but there are some crucial differences. Thus, according to Beck, risk is the defining characteristic of our age, and the heightened degree of risk reflexivity is the result of a greater number of risks being produced in the modern era (e.g. Beck 1992). People are more concerned about risk because they are being exposed to more risks. In contrast, Giddens has asserted that the number of risks is not actually any greater, but is simply *thought* to be greater, as people are now much more sensitive to risks (e.g. Giddens 1990, 1991). Thus, according to Giddens, modernity does not create risk and trust; it simply changes their nature. Both Beck and Giddens, however, have identified a greater awareness in lay people that the claims of experts are uncertain and need to be challenged. In addition, both have taken a weak social constructionist approach to risk, focusing their attention on how risk is generated and dealt with at the macro-structural level of society, as well as the political implications of this and the social conflicts that arise. However, both theorists have been criticized for portraying representations of modernity that are thought to be overly simplistic and for not having taken full account of the complexity of responses to expert knowledge (e.g. Lash 1993; Lupton 1999).

The governmentality perspective

While the risk society approach tends to take a weak social constructionist position, together with a critical structuralist perspective, advocates of the governmentality perspective have mostly adopted a strong version of social constructionism and a poststructuralist approach to power relations. According to the leading exponent of this third approach, Michel Foucault, risk strategies and discourses are a means of ordering the social and material worlds through methods of rationalization and calculation; that is, an attempt to render disorder and uncertainty more controllable (e.g. Foucault 1991). These strategies and discourses identify certain phenomena as being 'risky' and as requiring management by individuals or institutions. While the approach has received a lot of support, Foucault and others have been criticized for not paying sufficient attention to the question of how risk discourses and strategies operate or how they are negotiated or resisted by those who are the subject of them. Similarly, they have been criticized for their inadequate recognition of individual difference factors; that is, the ways in which people of different genders, ages and ethnicities may respond differently to the different discourses and strategies (e.g. Lupton 1999).

Risk assessment, perception, management and communication

This book is about risk communication, but in order to communicate effectively we need reliable information about risk, its extent and likely impact. We also need to know how this will be perceived by individuals and society. Finally, we need to understand how to manage or control risk, either as individuals or organizations. These are the main foci of interest for people working in the areas of risk assessment (measurement), risk perception and risk management respectively. We will look at each of these areas in turn, before considering the implications for risk communication.

Risk assessment

Risk assessment is concerned with the identification, characterization and quantification of risk. A major problem in risk assessment is how to get accurate and reliable measures of risks, particularly when levels of risk change over time and when risks are very small. This latter difficulty can lead to problems when trying to determine if a particular level of risk is acceptable. In the case of a new medicine, for example, at present only a relatively small number of patients need to take the drug before it is released onto the market. Thus, an adverse effect would need to be fairly common in order to become apparent in the trial. For many side-effects (that occur in, say, 1 per cent of people who take the medicine), over 30,000 people would need to take the drug before a statistical effect could be detected (and this is many more times the number who have to be exposed to the medicine before it can be released).

For many risks, however, the numbers are simply not available. As noted by the British Medical Association (1990), risks fall into three different classes:

1 Those for which plenty of statistics are available, and for which information on harm can be accurately collected.
2 Those for which some evidence may be available, but for which the relationship between hazard and harmful effect for any given individual cannot be estimated with certainty (e.g. cancer developing some years after exposure to radiation).
3 Risks of harmful events that have not yet happened and estimation of which is thus based on forecasts and probabilities (e.g. nuclear reactor failure in a power station).

A particular difficulty when assessing risk is that people modify both their levels of vigilance and their exposure to danger in response to their subjective perceptions of risk. It is now recognized, for example, that increasing the number of safety features in car design can lead some people to drive faster and take more risks. Thus, while car seatbelts have been shown to have a life-saving benefit if a driver is involved in an accident, there is also evidence that they can increase the chances of a driver being involved in a crash and can lead to increased pedestrian and cyclist injuries and fatalities as a result of motorists driving faster and taking more risks. Similarly, statistics show that fewer children get killed on the roads now than in the 1930s, but this does not necessarily mean that our roads are safer. As Hillman et al. (1990) noted, as traffic has grown and perceived danger increased, parents have responded by delaying the age at which they allow their children to cross roads, go out on bicycles or go to school alone. This means that accident rates cannot be used as objective measures of risk. If the rate is low, one cannot necessarily say that the level of risk is low, as a 'high' risk could have been perceived and avoided.

Another problem concerns reporting rates. Over the years, people have varied in their likelihood of reporting certain offences. For example, statistics show an increase in the number of sexual assaults, but we cannot tell from this whether more crimes are being committed or being *reported*. Confounds such as these create considerable difficulties for those trying to establish reliable measures of risk. In discussing this problem, Adams (1995) referred to what he terms the 'severity iceberg'. This is where the certainty in data increases as severity of injury increases, with fatality statistics being the most reliable, and minor injuries the least.

Risk perception

Whereas technologically sophisticated analysts employ risk assessment to evaluate hazards, the majority of people rely on intuitive risk judgements, typically referred to as risk perceptions. According to Pidgeon et al. (1992), risk perception involves people's beliefs, attitudes, judgements and feelings, as well as the wider social or cultural values and dispositions that people adopt towards hazards and their benefits. Risk perceptions are built up over time, are informed by personal experiences and social networks and are shaped by behavioural norms and media reporting.

One broad strategy for studying perceived risk has been to develop a taxonomy for hazards that can be used to understand and predict people's responses to risks. The most common approach has employed the 'psychometric paradigm', associated with Paul Slovic and colleagues (e.g. Slovic 1987). This approach uses psychophysical scaling and multivariate analysis techniques to produce quantitative representations or 'cognitive maps' of risk attitudes and perceptions. Thus, within the psychometric paradigm, people make quantitative judgements about the current and desired riskiness of different hazards.

The original impetus for the psychometric paradigm came from the pioneering work of Starr (1969), who attempted to develop a method for weighing technological risks against benefits in order to answer the question, 'How safe is safe?' After examining risk and benefit data for several industries and activities, Starr concluded that:

♦ acceptability of risk from an activity is roughly proportional to the third power of the benefits of that activity;
♦ the public will accept risks from voluntary activities (such as skiing) that are approximately 1000 times as great as they would from involuntary hazards that provide the same level of benefit.

More recent studies using the psychometric paradigm have shown that perceived risk is quantifiable and predictable, but is nevertheless inherently subjective. That is, it does not exist 'out there', independent of minds and cultures, waiting to be measured. Whereas Starr concluded that voluntariness of exposure was the key mediator of risk acceptance, Slovic and colleagues have argued that a number of other factors play a crucial role. Their expressed preference studies have shown that (perceived) characteristics such as familiarity, control, catastrophic potential, equity and level of knowledge also influence the relationship between perceived risk, perceived benefit and risk acceptance to differing degrees (e.g. Fischoff et al. 1978; Slovic et al. 1980).

One classic study by Slovic (1987), using the psychometric method, aimed to identify similarities and differences between the risk judgements of different groups of people. The study showed that risks were perceived differently by (and had a different meaning for) different groups, with the variance between experts and lay people being particularly apparent. For example, when experts judged risk, their assessment strongly related to objective risk indicators, whereas risk assessment by lay people was determined by other (more subjective) factors. Slovic used factor analysis to identify three dimensions underlying subjective risk perception. These were:

1 Dread risk – particularly where the consequences were potentially fatal and where there was a perceived lack of controllability.
2 Unknown risk – particularly where this had new or delayed consequences.
3 The number of people exposed to the risk, with concerns being greater when more people were involved.

More recent studies have confirmed the importance of these factors. After reviewing several such studies, Bennett (1998: 6) produced a list of 11 'fright factors'; that is, the attributes of risk most likely to invoke anxiety. He asserted that the risk is generally more worrying and less acceptable if:

♦ it is involuntary rather than voluntary;
♦ it threatens a form of death, illness or disease which arouses a particular dread;
♦ it damages identifiable victims;
♦ it is poorly understood by science;
♦ it is subject to contradictory statements from responsible sources or the same source;
♦ it is inescapable;
♦ it arises from an unfamiliar or novel source;
♦ it results from man-made rather than natural causes;
♦ it causes hidden and irreversible damage;
♦ it poses particular danger to small children, pregnant women or future generations;
♦ it is inequitably distributed.

Risk management

Risk management is the general term usually applied to the whole process of risk identification, estimation, evaluation, reduction and control. Petts (1992) suggested that the three primary goals of risk management are to control and reduce hazards to an acceptable level, to reduce the level of uncertainty in decision making about risks, and to increase public trust in risk matters. He distinguished between four main stages in the process, as follows:

1 Identifying the risks and any triggers.
2 Analysing the risks in terms of their frequency of occurrence, trends and impact.
3 Attempting to control the risks.
4 Costing the risks and controlling them.

The management of risk is a day to day activity for all of us. Managing risk does not necessarily entail reducing it, particularly at an individual level. A very common form of individual risk management is to buy insurance.

However, risk management tends to be more concerned with collective responses to risk than with individual risk-taking behaviour. It often takes place through direct government intervention, such as the introduction of laws and policies, and self-regulatory mechanisms in the private sector. Calman and Smith (2001) suggested that, in managing risk and forming policies, we need to address three key questions: What is the level of certainty of the risk and how strong is the evidence? Does the individual have any choice over whether he or she is subjected to the risk? What is the magnitude and acceptability of the risk being considered? Government and its various agencies are in a unique position of responsibility when it comes to regulating risks, setting guidelines for other authorities and informing people about risks. As Bennett and Calman (1999) have noted, at this level much of the debate about risk becomes interwoven with fundamental issues to do with power, information and the relationship between people and state.

Arguments about whether or not to introduce particular measures to reduce risk often centre on the cost and feasibility of the interventions. In general, however, as economic standards have increased, there has been pressure to reduce the level of risk that is publicly acceptable. Most activities, techniques and substances carry some risks, and to ban them all would be unfeasible and could result in an even higher level of harm than that created by the original risk (as is the case with vaccinations). In choosing between different alternatives, or in managing a situation, we need to find a level of risk that is deemed to be 'acceptable' or 'safe enough'. A working definition, in non-numeric terms, might be that 'a situation would be regarded as safe, and the associated hazards negligible, if reasonably informed and experienced people in fact disregard the risk' (British Medical Association 1990: 240). What people regard as safe enough will be affected by their confidence in their own, or others', ability to manage the risk in question.

The importance of trust

The management of risk clearly depends on people's perceptions and opinions, and the process necessarily entails an interaction and communication between groups or different stakeholders whose perceptions are inevitably different. Given that people, whether in groups or as individuals, tend to see things differently from each other, this creates a potential for misunderstanding and mistrust. Effective risk management relies heavily on trust, however. In recent years, many studies and surveys have documented the high level of distrust that we now have in many of the individuals, industries and institutions responsible for risk management (e.g. Slovic *et al.* 1991a; Frewer 1999). Who trusts whom, and why, are two of the most important questions in risk management and communication. If risk communicators and managers are to communicate effectively about the risks associated with particular hazards, it is essential to understand how people view, and trust, different sources of risk information. Hupcey *et al.* (2001: 285) defined trust as follows:

> trust emerges from the identification of a need that cannot be met without the assistance of another and some assessment of the risk involved in relying on the other to meet this need. Trust is a willing dependency on another's actions, but is limited to the area of need and is subject to overt and covert testing. The outcome of trust is an evaluation of the congruence between expectations of the trusted person and actions.

Research has shown that trust is multifaceted rather than one-dimensional, with relevant factors including perceived competence, objectivity, fairness and consistency. Different sources often score differently on these dimensions and across different issues (Frewer 1999). Renn and Levine (1991) similarly distinguished between five source characteristics that affect trust, these being: perceived competence, objectivity, fairness, consistency and faith. More recently, Frewer (2003) identified two major dimensions that have emerged from the social psychological literature as being important in determining trust: competence and honesty. According to Frewer, trust appears to be linked to perceptions of accuracy, knowledge and concern with public welfare. Distrust is associated with perceptions of deliberate distortion of information, being biased and having been proven wrong in the past.

Trust is clearly a function of both care and competence and is also integral to credibility (a key consideration for whether a message is believed and acted on). The professional values of competence, expertise, honesty and commitment are therefore all relevant to communicating risk. Getting the facts right and conveying them in an understandable way is not enough (Edwards 2003). As Paling (2003) pointed out, the most powerful precursor for effective risk communication in health is for the doctor to strive to display both competence and a caring approach. High competence and care lead to trust, whereas low competence and care lead to distrust. Both factors are seen as being necessary; high competence and a low caring approach may lead to respect, and low competence and a high caring approach may lead to affection, but neither combination will result in trust.

Evidence has shown that, in the absence of trust, risk messages may be ignored. However, we also know that trust is very fragile; it is created slowly but can be destroyed in an instant. Once trust is lost it takes a long time to rebuild and sometimes never can be. In relation to this, Slovic (2000) referred to his 'asymmetry principle', which involves the following four elements:

1 Negative (trust destroying) events are more visible than positive (trust-building) events.
2 When events come to our notice, negative events carry more weight.

3 Sources of bad news seem to be more credible than sources of good news.
4 Distrust, once initiated, tends to reinforce and perpetuate itself.

Thus it is essential for those involved in risk management and communication to use 'trusted' sources of information where possible, and to try to ensure that trust in those sources is maintained.

We have seen earlier that people's health beliefs can be adversely affected by inaccuracies in their perceptions of risk. It is also the case that people can be 'hurt' by inaccuracies in what various risk managers believe about those perceptions (Fischoff *et al.* 1993). In the health arena, such risk managers include doctors, nurses, hospital administrators, public health authorities and various government and regulatory officials. If people's understanding is overestimated, then they may be thrust into situations that they are ill-equipped to handle. If, on the other hand, their level of understanding is underestimated, then people may become disenfranchised from decisions that they could and should make, leading to a loss of empowerment.

Social amplification of risk

Another feature of risk that needs to be acknowledged in relation to effective management is that hazardous events often have impacts that extend far beyond any direct harmful effects and may include a number of indirect costs (e.g. to government or private organizations) that can far exceed any direct costs. These 'ripple' effects are captured in Kasperson *et al.*'s (1988) social amplification model (see Figure 2.1). The model focuses on the interaction of hazard-driven events with psychological, social, institutional and cultural processes, resulting in the amplification and attenuation of individual and social perceptions of risk and the shaping of risk behaviour. According to the social amplification model, the process starts with recognition of an adverse effect, which is then communicated. An example might be the CSM's warning about the doubled risk of thrombosis with third generation oral contraceptives (see Chapter 1).

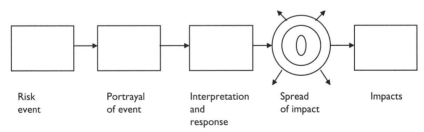

| Risk event | Portrayal of event | Interpretation and response | Spread of impact | Impacts |

Figure 2.1   A simplified version of Kasperson *et al.*'s (1988) social amplification model

Individuals, groups and institutions collect and respond to risk information and act as amplification stations through behavioural responses and communication. In relation to the 'pill scare', amplification stations included individuals, health professionals and the media. The behavioural patterns in turn generate secondary social or economic consequences that can extend far beyond direct harm to humans or the environment. Thus, following the 'pill scare', there was an increased number of unwanted pregnancies and terminations which then had additional knock-on effects on families, the health care system and pharmaceutical companies. Clearly, therefore, risk communicators and managers must look beyond the immediate effects of any action or communication to consider a much broader range of unfolding indirect effects, and must extend the time period over which they assess the effects of particular risks.

Risk communication

Difficulties in assessment, perception and management of risk all have implications for risk communication. If we do not have accurate information about the 'real' level of risk in most situations, if people perceive risk differently and vary in what they believe to be an appropriate balance between risk and reward, and if people have a tendency not to trust the information that they are given by government and certain official bodies, then determining what information to present to them, and in what form, is far from straightforward. However, as Jungermann (1997) noted, informing people about risks has become a political necessity as well as a moral obligation. It is not something that we can simply opt out of.

Defining risk communication

Risk communication can be defined as 'communication with individuals (not necessarily face-to-face) which addresses knowledge, perceptions, attitudes and behaviour relating to risk' (Edwards and Bastian 2001: 147). Covello (1991) distinguished between four areas in which risk communication is applied: informing and education; stimulating behavioural change and taking protective measures; issuing of disaster warnings and emergency information; and exchange of information and a common approach to risk issues. Similarly, Green et al. (1999: 59) noted that risk communication can serve a number of purposes ranging from the development of risk management policies to informing people about the various risks to which they are exposed. Thus, according to these writers, risk communication includes:

♦ statutory requirements to inform the public and other bodies about certain large-scale technological risks;
♦ communication of technical information between scientists, policy makers and risk managers to inform decision making;

- ◆ communication between all stakeholder groups to inform decision making;
- ◆ provision of information which allows individuals to make informed decisions about whether to accept a risk or not, and to take certain risk-reducing actions.

Given this range, it seems likely that different strategies of risk communication will be more appropriate for different goals. A simple vivid risk message, for instance, might be best for raising awareness, while stakeholder participation methods might be better for stimulating behavioural change (Bier 2001). Similarly, what we might consider to be appropriate measures of success will vary depending on the purpose of the communication and the intended audience.

Clearly, risk communication can take many different forms and comprise many issues. Thus, we could learn about a particular risk through a major government public education campaign, a TV documentary or newspaper account, from a consultation with a doctor, from warnings on medication or food products and so on. A particular risk message might be aimed at an individual (as in a doctor–patient consultation or a genetic counselling session) or at a wider section of the general population as part of a public health or health promotion campaign (see Chapter 5). The impact of the communication will depend on the content and form of presentation of the message, its source and the characteristics of the particular target audience.

In general, risk communication involves determining who conveys what, to whom, how and with what effect. Risk communication can be considered to be effective if it alerts the target audience as to what is hazardous, the extent of the danger and what should be done as a result. In relation to human health, effective communications should help people to reduce their health risks or to get greater benefit in return for any risks that they decide to take. More specifically, Edwards (2003) recommended that risk communications should be simply worded, relevant and responsive to the needs and values of individual patients. There should be a two-way exchange of opinions and values as well as information seeking to maximize trust and support. Similarly, Alaszewski and Horlick-Jones (2003) suggested that, to improve risk communications with patients, doctors need to build up relationships of trust, be aware of the multiple and conflicting sources of risk information that patients access, and be sensitive to the psychological and social factors that influence the ways in which patients respond to risk information.

Such factors are important as ineffective risk communications can lead to inappropriate decisions by omitting important information or failing to correct misconceptions. In addition, they can create confusion by emphasizing irrelevant information and can result in a loss of trust in the communicator or the source of the message content. By causing either complacency or unwarranted alarm, inappropriate risk messages can have a

more serious adverse effect on public health outcomes than the risks that
they attempt to address, as was seen in the 1995 'pill scare'. As noted by
Fischoff *et al.* (1993), it is no more acceptable to release an untested risk
communication than an untested drug.

The complexities of risk communication

Communication of risk is clearly complex and multifaceted. Calman (2002)
identified three factors that are relevant in risk communication: the
certainty of the risk (i.e. the evidence base); the level of risk (e.g. high or
low); and the effect of the risk on the individual or population. As Calman
noted, risks can range from being biologically plausible but with there being
no level of certainty in relation to their size or effect, to clearly identifiable
risks with known levels and effects. Clearly, communication will be much
more problematic in the former case, although, as Calman pointed out, even
in the latter case, in most situations, the particular effects on any individual
still remain uncertain.

The mass media play an important role in shaping perceptions of risk. As
Paling (2003) argued, although experts can measure risk and (attempt to)
communicate their measurements to the public, the information is usually
filtered through various media, which affects its interpretation by social
groups and individuals. The influence of the media can be viewed as being
positive or negative depending on the particular circumstances. In the case
of the 1995 'pill scare' it is usually acknowledged that the media's influence
was primarily detrimental, as most of the coverage was unbalanced and
sensationalist, increasing alarm in many women. However, as Bennett
(1998) has noted, the media does not usually create public interest. Rather,
they simply amplify (albeit sometimes to a considerable degree) existing
public interest in particular 'forms of mishap'. Thus, public and media
interest reinforce each other. Bennett identified a number of 'media
triggers' that determine the extent of coverage that is given to a particular
issue. These include questions of blame, alleged secrets or cover-ups,
human interest, links with high-profile issues or personalities, the existence
of conflict and the fact that many people are, or could be, affected by the risk
in question.

As Jungermann (1997) has noted, risk communicators face many
problems which stem from technical, scientific, cognitive and social limitations that relate to the various components of the risk communication
process. For example, problems can arise in relation to the source of the
communication, the message itself, the channel by which it is communicated and the receiver of the message. It is not surprising, therefore, that
risk communication is often a contentious process. As Bennett and Calman
(1999: v) pointed out, from one point of view the temptation is to see the
public, egged on by the media, as 'misunderstanding perfectly sensible
information and advice'. This can be illustrated by a former UK Secretary
of State for Health who when commenting on consumer reactions to the

BSE crisis stated that 'we were dealing with mad consumers rather than mad cows' (McKechnie and Davies 1999: 178). From the other point of view, however, authorities are often seen to be 'withholding or obfuscating vital pieces of the picture and to be impervious to perfectly reasonable public concerns' (Bennett and Calman 1999: v). Establishing an effective middle ground is not easy. However, it is clear that the 'old fashioned view of risk communication as a one way process of drip feeding expert knowledge on to a supposedly grateful public' will no longer do (Bennett and Calman 1999: vi).

Doing an effective job of risk communication often means finding comprehensible ways of presenting complex material that is clouded by uncertainty and is inherently difficult to understand. As noted by Calman *et al.* (1999), we live in increasingly challenging times in terms of risk communication. In particular, new challenges are being raised by advances in technology that are giving rise to new risks, and by advances in science that are allowing us to identify low-level risks that already existed but were not previously acknowledged. Risk communicators must be fully aware of the strengths and limits of the methods used to generate the information they are attempting to convey to the public. In particular, communicators need to understand that risk assessments are often constructed from theoretical models that are based on assumptions and subjective judgements. If these assumptions and judgements are deficient then the resulting estimates may be inaccurate, or at least different from those of the communicators. In conjunction with this, they also have to acknowledge that there are limitations in public understanding. As we will see in the next chapter, people's perceptions of risk are often inaccurate. Furthermore, risk information may frighten and frustrate the public. Evidence has shown that strong beliefs are particularly difficult to modify and that, when people do not hold strong beliefs, their views and judgements can be significantly influenced by the particular ways in which information is presented. This presents risk communicators with a considerable challenge. Sir Kenneth Calman, former Chief Medical Officer in the UK, proposed that the main purpose of risk communication is to produce an informed public that is involved, reasonable, thoughtful and collaborative (e.g. Calman *et al.* 1999). However, the chapters that follow show that producing such an informed public is by no means a straightforward or easy task.

Communicating probabilistic information

We have seen in the previous chapter that in order to make effective decisions, people need to understand the risks and benefits associated with the different options that they face. They also need to understand the limits of their knowledge, as well as the limits of any 'expert' advice that they are given. This means that people not only need to be given reliable information about risks and benefits, but they also need to be able to understand the information and its limitations so that they can use it effectively. However, as we will see in the sections that follow, there is now a firm body of evidence showing that many people are subject to various cognitive difficulties when interpreting probabilistic information. Furthermore, we are all prone to a range of cognitive biases, and our interpretation of risk information is often influenced by the particular way in which it is presented to us. Finally, we will see that a number of emotional and affective factors will also play a role in how we interpret and respond to particular risk communications.

Cognitive biases and heuristics

In order to choose effectively between different options, the decision maker has to make judgements about, and compare, the probability of different outcomes. There are various normative statistical methods for doing this which should produce the 'correct answer'. However, a large body of work, primarily associated with Amos Tversky and Daniel Kahneman, has shown that, in many everyday situations, people tend to use simpler 'short-cut heuristics' or 'rules of thumb' (see Tversky and Kahneman 1974 for an overview). Such heuristics frequently lead to the correct answer but are sometimes associated with systematic errors or biases. The two heuristics identified by Tversky and Kahneman that have received the most attention in the literature are 'representativeness' and 'availability' (for a recent collection of papers see Gilovitch *et al.* 2002).

Representativeness

The representativeness heuristic is studied in situations in which people are asked to judge the probability that an object or event belongs to a particular class. For example, a person might be given the description of an individual and asked to estimate the probability that this individual has a certain occupation. According to Tversky and Kahneman (e.g. 1974), events that are representative or typical of a class are assigned a high probability of occurrence. If an event is highly similar to most of the others in a population then it is considered to be representative. The problem with using this heuristic is that representativeness does not take account of certain key types of information, such as relative sample size or underlying base rates, that are known to influence the outcome. A classic experiment showing how use of heuristics leads people to ignore base rates was reported by Kahneman and Tversky in 1973. Participants in their study were presented with brief personality sketches and were told that the descriptions were drawn at random from a sample of either 70 engineers and 30 lawyers, or 30 engineers and 70 lawyers (i.e. people were given different base rates of lawyers and engineers in the population). So, for example, they were presented with a description such as the following:

> Jack is a 45-year-old man. He is married and has four children. He is generally conservative, careful and ambitious. He shows no interest in political and social issues and spends most of his free time on his many hobbies, which include home carpentry, sailing and mathematical puzzles.

The participants decided that there was a 90 per cent chance that Jack was an engineer, regardless of the underlying base rate (i.e. 70 or 30 engineers out of 100). It cannot be argued, however, that they were simply unable to utilize the base rate information. When given a completely neutral personality sketch they did take full account of the base rate information that was provided and responded in line with this.

Another problem that arises as a result of use of the 'representativeness' heuristic is that people often show misconceptions of chance. Thus, they expect that the essential characteristics of a process will be represented not only in the entire sequence but also locally in each of its parts. A well-known consequence of this is the phenomenon known as 'gambler's fallacy'. For example, after observing a long run of red on the roulette wheel, most people believe that the probability of the wheel landing on black on the next spin is much greater than the probability of it landing on red (even though the actual likelihood is equal in the two cases). People believe that the occurrence of black would result in a more 'representative' series. In other words, chance is viewed as a self-correcting process, even in the short term. Similarly, in relation to coin tosses, people believe that a sequence such as HTHHTH is more likely to occur (i.e. is more representative) than either HHHTTT or HTHHHH (where H stands for heads and T for tails), even though the three have equal probabilities of occurrence. The latter two sequences are viewed as being 'not random' or 'unfair', respectively, as people expect 'randomness' to operate even in such short sequences.

Availability

This second heuristic involves estimating the frequencies of events on the basis of how easy or difficult it is to bring particular instances to mind. For example, Tversky and Kahneman (1974) asked people the following question: 'If a word of three letters or more is sampled from an English text, is it more likely that the word starts with the letter "r" or has "r" as its third letter?' They found that the majority of participants believed that a word starting with 'r' was more likely, whereas in reality the reverse is the case. According to Tversky and Kahneman, people respond incorrectly because words beginning with the letter 'r' can be more easily retrieved from memory (i.e. they are more available) than words that have 'r' as their third letter.

Studies have also shown that availability can be based on actual frequency of occurrence, in that we tend to recall those things that have been encountered most frequently in the past. However, such judgements are often influenced by the relative salience of instances. A classic experiment by Lichtenstein et al. (1978) showed that causes of death that attract more publicity (e.g. murder) are judged more likely to occur than those that attract less publicity (e.g. suicide or certain types of cancer), contrary to the true state of affairs.

However, Schwartz and Vaughn (2002) have argued that many of the classic studies on availability are ambiguous with regard to the underlying process. Thus in the case of the letter 'r' experiment, people's judgements could be based on either the degree of 'ease of memory recall' or the actual 'content' of the recall (i.e. the number of words that they bring to mind in the two cases). Schwartz and Vaughn cited a number of studies which show that the particular source of information adopted when making a judgement will depend on the details of the context and individual difference factors. For example, Rothman and Schwartz (1998) found that male undergraduates with a family history of heart disease were more likely to rely on content of recall when judging vulnerability to a heart attack, whereas those without such a family history were more likely to rely on ease of recall.

Other cognitive biases

Two other heuristics that have received less research and attention than representativeness and availability are 'anchoring and adjustment' and 'numerosity'. Anchoring applies in situations where people's judgements are influenced by a particular 'anchor' that they are given. They then make adjustments from this starting value when assessing probabilities (Tversky and Kahneman 1974). For example, in the Lichtenstein *et al.* (1978) study, people's estimates of the number of murders or suicides per year were influenced by an example estimate that they were given (either 50,000 annual deaths in motor accidents or 1000 deaths by electrocution). People judged the number of murders to be larger if they were given a large example estimate (i.e. a larger anchor).

The numerosity heuristic was introduced by Pelham *et al.* (1994). They found that judgements of quantity were influenced by the number of items making up the total quantity. Thus, people judged the area of a circle to be larger when it was cut into many pieces, like a pizza. Pelham *et al.* pointed to many similar findings in the animal learning literature, and drew on evolutionary principles to support their case for the numerosity effect being a basic cognitive heuristic.

A critical perspective

There is now considerable evidence that many of our everyday judgements are influenced by biases such as representativeness and availability. However, some researchers have argued that the use of heuristics may not be as pervasive as Tversky and Kahneman and others have claimed. For example, Pollard and Evans (1983) pointed out that many of the problems employed by Kahneman and Tversky to demonstrate the use of heuristics were linguistically complex, and this may have confused participants. One of the strongest critiques, however, has come from Gerd Gigerenzer and colleagues. In particular, Gigerenzer and Goldstein (1996) have argued that errors are less prevalent if the problems are recast in terms of frequencies rather than as probabilities. In a number of experimental studies Gigerenzer has shown that the 'biasing' effects of heuristics disappear when frequency information is provided (e.g. Hoffrage and Gigerenzer 1998; Hoffrage *et al.* 2000). Thus, for example, Hoffrage *et al.* (2000) found that doctors were able to take full account of base rate information rather than being biased by 'representativeness' when problems were recast in terms of frequencies rather than percentages. Only 1 of 24 doctors produced the correct answer in the latter case, compared with 16 out of 24 in the former (see also Cosmides and Tooby 1996). As we will see in the next sections, both Gigerenzer, and Cosmides and Tooby, have drawn on evolutionary principles to support their arguments.

Difficulties with presenting and interpreting probability information

In addition to being susceptible to various cognitive biases, our risk percep- tions can be adversely affected by basic cognitive limitations. A number of studies have shown that many people have difficulty understanding relatively simple numerical information. Schwartz *et al.* (1997), for example, found that only 16 per cent of 500 women were able to answer three simple numeracy questions (e.g. converting percentages into proportions and vice versa) correctly. Similar results were reported by Lipkus *et al.* (2001) and by Bynner and Parsons (1997) in their study of the 1958 birth cohort group. Such difficulties are not just limited to members of the general population with poorer educational backgrounds. Sheridan and Pignone (2002) found similar difficulties in a sample of medical students.

The trouble with percentages

We saw in Chapter 1 that Patricia Hewitt was quoted in the *Independent* newspaper in November 2002 as saying that 'fifty per cent of the public doesn't actually know what 50% means'. Although this is likely to be an exaggeration, there is considerable evidence that many people have dif- ficulty interpreting percentages. In Chapter 1, we referred to a study show- ing that over a third of a sample of 1000 Germans were unable to interpret the term '40 per cent' correctly, mistakenly believing that it meant one in four or every fortieth person, rather than four out of every ten people (Gigerenzer 2002).

Part of the difficulty is that percentages are often ambiguous. Thus, the statement 'there is a 40 per cent chance that it will snow tomorrow' could be interpreted to mean that it will snow 40 per cent of the time, that it will snow in 40 per cent of the area or that it will snow on 40 per cent of days like tomorrow. As Gigerenzer (2002) pointed out, one difficulty is that the reference class is often unclear when single event probabilities are described as percentages. Thus, he referred to a psychiatrist friend who used to tell his patients that there was a 30 to 50 per cent chance of developing a sexual problem, such as impotence, from taking Prozac. The psychiatrist subsequently found out that many patients would not take the drug as they interpreted the statement to mean that if they did take it, something would go wrong on 30 to 50 per cent of occasions, rather than to mean that 30 to 50 per cent of people would be afflicted.

Presenting probabilities as frequencies

Several researchers, but most notably Gerd Gigerenzer, have argued that many of the above difficulties go away if probabilities are presented as frequencies rather than as percentages. In terms of the above example, the psychiatrist found that people became more willing to take Prozac once he started to explain that out of every ten people given the drug, three to five experience a sexual problem. According to Gigerenzer (2002), the benefit of using frequencies rather than percentages becomes even more apparent with more complex information, as can be seen in the following example:

> The probability that a woman of age 40 has breast cancer is about 1 per cent. If she has breast cancer, the probability that she tests positive on a screening mammogram is 90 per cent. If she does not have breast cancer, the probability that she nevertheless tests positive is 9 per cent. What are the chances that a woman who tests positive actually has breast cancer?
>
> (Gigerenzer 2002: 41)

Most people find the above problem confusing. Many believe that the answer is 90 per cent, but are not very confident that they are correct. Now read the same problem presented using natural frequencies:

> Think of 100 women. One has breast cancer, and she will probably test positive. Of the 99 who do not have breast cancer, 9 will also test positive. Thus a total of 10 women will test positive. How many of those who test positive actually have breast cancer?
>
> (Gigerenzer 2002: 42)

People find that it is easier to see that only one woman out of every ten who tests positive will actually have cancer; that is, the probability is 10 per cent not 90 per cent. In recent years, a number of experimental studies have provided evidence to confirm that many people perform better when making judgements using frequency information than percentages (e.g. Cosmides and Tooby 1996; Hoffrage and Gigerenzer 1998, 2000; Brase 2002). Cosmides and Tooby (1996), for example, presented people with various frequentist versions of diagnosis problems, similar to the one just described, and found that they took full account of the base rate information that was provided. When the problems were presented using percentages, people ignored this information and overly weighted the test information. Similarly, Hoffrage et al. (2000) presented 96 advanced medical students with four realistic medical diagnosis tasks (two of which were described using probabilities and two using frequencies). They found that significantly more students correctly inferred the likelihood of having the disease given a positive test result when the statistics were communicated using natural frequencies. More recently, Brase (2002) has shown that simple frequencies, based on small reference classes (e.g. 1 in 3) were perceived as clearer than percentages (e.g. 33 per cent) and single event probabilities (e.g. 0.33). In addition, he found that absolute frequencies were relatively more persuasive for smaller magnitudes (e.g. 2.7 million) but less persuasive for larger magnitudes (e.g. 267 million).

It is not just lay people and students who have difficulty reasoning with probabilities. In the context of medical diagnosis, Eddy (1982) found that experienced doctors made similar errors to those made by non-medically qualified people. More recently, Hoffrage and Gigerenzer (1998) tested 48 physicians, with an average of 14 years experience, on a diagnosis problem similar to that shown above. When the problem was presented using percentages, they found enormous variation in the physicians' responses, which ranged from 10 to 90 per cent (with an average of 70 per cent). Only two doctors produced the correct answer. However, when the same problem was presented using natural frequencies there was much less variance, with the majority producing the correct answer or close to it. Only five of the doctors thought that the probability of breast cancer given a positive mammography was greater than 50 per cent.

Gigerenzer (2002) asserted that representing information in terms of frequencies rather than probabilities is beneficial for two reasons. The first is computational simplicity, in that natural frequencies actually do part of the computation that has to be done mentally with probabilistic forms of presentation. The second reason is evolutionary and developmental primacy. Gigerenzer argued that our minds are adapted to natural frequencies because natural frequencies result from natural sampling, the process by which humans (and animals) have encountered information about risks during most of their evolution. Cosmides and Tooby (1996) similarly drew on evolutionary arguments to explain their findings.

Degrees of belief

In addition to representing probabilistic information as logical probabilities or frequencies, a third option is a form of representation based on degrees of belief (Baron 1994). The idea of probability as degree of belief allows for more of a role for individual judgement. In determining horse race odds, for example, bookmakers will take account of factors such as the previous form of the horse and jockey, the horse's breeding, the condition of the racecourse and so on. Although degrees of belief can be represented as numerical probabilities (and indeed are by bookmakers), a more natural form of representation involves the use of verbal frequency labels.

Interpretation of verbal probability expressions

Over the past 30 years, a large body of research has looked at how people interpret common verbal probability terms such as 'likely' or 'rare'. Except in situations where the odds are objectively measurable, many people (including experts in a variety of domains) feel more at ease using verbal probability expressions than numbers (see e.g. Renooij and Witteman 1999). However, several studies have shown a paradoxical effect in that, although most people prefer to use verbal expressions to convey risks, they like to receive risk information in the form of numerical probabilities (see e.g. Erev and Cohen 1990; Wallsten *et al.* 1993). To explain this effect, Fox and Irwin (1998) suggested that quantitative expressions are perceived by the speaker to be unnaturally precise, and the vagueness inherent in qualitative statements helps to capture their second order uncertainty (see also Wallsten and Budescu 1990). Timmermans (1994) also noted that many doctors are reluctant to use numerical expressions because they imply more precision than is usually warranted by the available evidence.

One major problem with using verbal labels, however, is that there is considerable variance in terms of how they are interpreted. Toogood (1980), for example, asked people to give the occurrence rates associated with nine frequency adverbs, ranging from 'always' to 'never', and found that participants associated radically different frequencies with the same word. For instance, interpretations of the term 'often' ranged from 28 to 92 per cent. Although subsequent studies have shown that interpretation is typically influenced by factors such as context and the experience level of the person concerned, it is still the case that large differences remain, even when considering only a single context and a more limited sample. In a medical context, for example, Bryant and Norman (1980) found that physicians' interpretations of the term 'likely' ranged from 25 to 75 per cent. More recently, Timmermans (1994) reported that interpretations of the term 'very likely' ranged from 30 to 90 per cent, even when presented in a restricted medical context. Similarly, Mazur and Merz (1994) found a comparable degree of diversity in patients' interpretations of the word 'rare'.

Despite difficulties such as these, several researchers have nevertheless argued that there are considerable advantages in using verbal labels. Weber and Hilton (1990), for example, proposed that an advantage of verbal probability expressions is that they not only convey a level of uncertainty, but they also imply a certain amount of imprecision about that level. In line with this, Renooij and Witteman (1999) suggested that verbal expressions are perceived as more natural, easier to understand and communicate and better suited to conveying the vagueness of one's opinions. Similarly, Windschitl and Wells (1996) advocated that verbal descriptions of uncertainty have the advantage that they allow for more associative and intuitive thinking. They pointed out that there are many situations in which human decisions and behaviours are not based on deliberate and rule-based thinking, and that the use of numerical descriptions may well misrepresent how individuals think about uncertainty in such situations. Windschitl and Wells reported three experiments which showed that, relative to numerical values, verbal descriptors were more sensitive to manipulations of context and framing, and were better predictors of people's preferences and behavioural intentions.

Differences between experts and novices

Some researchers have argued that physicians and patients differ in their interpretations of verbal probability terms, but the available evidence is far from conclusive. For instance, although Nakao and Axelrod (1983) and Ohnishi *et al.* (2002) reported more consensus among doctors than lay people in their numerical interpretations of a set of verbal descriptors, Kong *et al.* (1986) found no such difference. Similarly, Timmermans (1994) found no effect of level of expertise in the interpretations of junior, intermediate and senior doctors. After reviewing a large number of studies on how experts assess risks, Rowe and Wright (2001) concluded that it is not possible to draw any firm conclusions about expert-lay differences in the quality or nature of such risk judgements. Although many of the studies they reviewed showed expert assessments of risk to be lower than those of lay people, the majority of the studies did not actually assess the veracity of the judgements. Furthermore, Rowe and Wright noted a number of methodological problems with the studies including several potential confounding factors, such as the gender and level of education of the participants.

Effects of context

Evidence has consistently shown, however, that people's interpretations are influenced by the particular context in which the judgement is made. As noted by Parducci (1968), a student may think that if her contraceptives failed on 5 per cent of occasions this would be 'often', whereas if she were absent from 5 per cent of her classes this would be 'almost never'. Parducci's claims have been backed up by findings from a number of empirical studies. Wallsten *et al.* (1986), for instance, found that lower numerical equivalents were assigned to the same verbal expressions when applied to events that were assumed to happen only rarely, as opposed to more frequently (such as the chance of snow falling in North Carolina in October rather than in December). Similar findings were reported by Weber and Hilton (1990), who showed that probability judgements were influenced by severity of outcome (e.g. 'likely' death as opposed to 'likely' injury, with lower estimates being given for the more serious outcomes). In the medical context, Merz *et al.* (1991) reviewed over 450 information consent decisions and found that verbal expressions of probability were influenced by the severity of the consequences.

More generally, Fox and Irwin (1998) have proposed that the social, informational, motivational and discourse context in which beliefs are constructed and statements are formulated provides a myriad of additional cues that influence what is expressed by speakers and what is understood by listeners. Thus, context can be provided by the characteristics of the stimulus domain, the perceiver's knowledge and experience, the goal of the communication, the way the information is framed, the presence of multiple alternatives or the way that probabilities are presented. In addition, Moxey and Sandford (1993) found that the interpretation of natural language quantifiers depends, in part, on one's prior expectations about what the proportions being described might be. Thus, if an event has a high base rate probability, such as the number of people who enjoy parties, then the value assigned to the quantifier 'many' is higher than it is for a low base rate expectation, such as the number of doctors in a hospital who are female. Similar effects were subsequently found with commonplace risk expressions, such as 'negligible risk', 'small risk' and 'significant risk' (Moxey and Sandford 2000).

As we will see in Chapter 6, studies in our own laboratory have shown that people vary in their interpretation of European Commission (EC) recommended verbal descriptors, such as 'common', depending on whether they are used to describe mild or severe side-effects, and whether the medicine in question is being prescribed for an adult or a 1-year-old child (Berry in press). A particularly interesting finding was reported by Abramsky and Fletcher (2002) who investigated how health professionals and lay people perceive words commonly used in prenatal diagnosis counselling. They found that the vast majority of the sample (88 per cent) felt that being told of a '*rare* chromosome abnormality' in a baby was con-siderably more worrying than being told of a '*common* chromosome abnormality'.

Interestingly, several investigators have shown that numerical probability expressions are not immune to context effects. Windschitl and Weber (1999), for example, found that when people were told that a woman had a 30 per cent chance of developing malaria on an upcoming trip, their degree of certainty as to whether or not she would develop the disease varied according to whether the trip was to India or to Hawaii. Similarly, Windschitl *et al.* (2002) found that people judged a target group to be more vulnerable to a disease when the prevalence rate for a context group was low rather than high, and Flugstad and Windschitl (2003) reported that people's judgements were also influenced by the reasons that experts gave to justify their estimates.

Other influences on the way we interpret risk information

Different numerical formats

Many people not only have difficulty understanding percentages, and are inconsistent in their interpretation of verbal probability labels, but their judgements can also be influenced by the particular way in which numbers are presented. Halpern *et al.* (1989: 253), for example, provided participants with statistical information about the chances of death due to circulatory problems in oral contraceptive users. They used six different presentation formats, as follows:

♦ 99,991.7 out of 100,000 will not die
♦ 0.0083 per cent probability of dying
♦ 1 in 12,000 die
♦ 8.3 in 100,000 die
♦ 4.15 times greater risk of death
♦ 415 per cent greater risk of death

They found that the different formats resulted in very different judgements of probability of death. For example, the participants rated the risk to be much higher when told that there was a 415 per cent greater risk of death than when told that the risk was 4.15 times higher. More recently, Yamagishi (1997) presented people with two different statements about a certain type of cancer and asked them which they judged to be more risky:

♦ kills 1286 out of 10,000 people
♦ kills 24.14 out of 100 people

The first statement was judged as being much more risky even though the level of risk described in the second is actually twice as high. Thus, people's judgements are overly influenced by the number of people killed, and they take insufficient account of the size of the overall sample under consideration.

The fact that people can be misled by varying sizes of sample or population has implications for presenting probability information in terms of '1 in X' frequency expressions. Studies have shown that people sometimes judge a '1 in 214' risk to be smaller (i.e. safer) than a '1 in 21,400' risk.

Relative and absolute forms of presentation

Another way in which judgements can be affected by different presentation formats, and one that has received considerable attention in recent years, is whether risk levels are described in absolute or relative terms. Absolute risk reduction can be thought of as the difference between risk of an event in a control group and risk of an event in a treatment group. In contrast, relative risk is the ratio of risks of the treatment group and control group. The relative risk reduction is derived from the relative risk by subtracting it from 'one' (Schechtman 2002).

Many studies have shown that giving people information about relative risk reductions can have more influence on their judgements and be more likely to lead to the uptake of particular behaviours than giving them information about absolute risk reductions. This can be illustrated as follows: if the chance of having a disease is 10 per cent and this reduces to

5 per cent when a person takes a certain drug, then this can be thought of as an absolute risk reduction of 5 per cent or as a relative risk reduction of 50 per cent. Not surprisingly, people are often very influenced by such relative descriptions. Malenka *et al.* (1993), for instance, reported that choice of medication was influenced by whether the reported benefit from taking the medicine was presented in relative or absolute terms. Nearly 80 per cent of their participants opted for the medication that was presented with information about relative risk benefits compared with 20 per cent for the medicine that was presented with information about absolute risk benefits. Similarly, Hux and Naylor (1995) found that more than twice as many patients opted to undergo lipid lowering therapy when informed of the relative risk reduction compared with the absolute risk reduction. In addition, doctors have been shown to be more likely to prescribe particular medicines if the benefits are described in relative rather than in absolute terms (see e.g. Forrow *et al.* 1992; Lacy *et al.* 2001; Nexoe *et al.* 2002), and health policy makers have been shown to be more willing to purchase various health services (such as cardiac rehabilitation) if risk reductions are communicated in relative terms (Fahey *et al.* 1995).

Such striking differences are not just confined to experimental studies but have also been observed in relation to everyday health behaviours. For example, it is known that the risk of developing breast cancer after five years of (oestrogen only) hormone replacement therapy (HRT) increases by 30 per cent. When patients are given this information by their doctor, they are often alarmed by the level of risk and frequently decide not to have the therapy. However, the absolute level of risk involved is actually rather low (10 per cent). When women are given the same information in absolute terms (i.e. they are informed that the risk with HRT rises from 10 per cent to 13 per cent), it has been found that they are much more likely to undergo the treatment.

As we saw in Chapter 1, an even more striking effect of relative risk presentations was observed in relation to the 1995 'pill scare', which was provoked by warnings of an almost doubled risk of thrombosis for users of third generation oral contraceptives. The scare received considerable media attention and resulted in many women stopping taking the pill, together with a sharp rise in unwanted pregnancies and terminations. Again, however, the absolute level of risk involved was very low. Use of third generation oral contraceptives only increased the risk from around 15 cases per annum per 100,000 pill users to around 25 cases. The crucial point, however, is that the risk in pregnancy is actually four to five times higher. So, telling women about the risk of thrombosis from taking the pill led to an increase in pregnancies, which then put women at even greater risk. Following the scare, the CSM published a recommended wording describing the levels of risk of thrombosis associated with pill use and pregnancy, to be used on all information leaflets distributed with the contraceptives. Unfortunately, however, they did not adequately evaluate women's understanding of the recommended wording. We recently carried out an evaluation of this wording and found that less than 12 per cent of women in higher education fully understood, and could make simple inferences from, the text (Berry *et al.* 2002c). The finding is particularly worrying as the wording is currently given to millions of women each year, many of whom are less well educated than the people in our study.

The detrimental effects of the original 'pill scare' were very much exacerbated by unbalanced media reporting, with the majority of accounts emphasizing the doubling of risk associated with third generation contraceptives, and failing to mention the absolute levels of risk involved. Such unbalanced reporting appears to be fairly widespread. Moynihan *et al.* (2000) analysed 207 news media stories (relating to three different drugs) that appeared between 1994 and 1998, and found that the majority included inadequate or incomplete information about the risks, benefits and costs of the medicines. Worryingly, 83 per cent reported relative risk (or benefits) only, with the remainder reporting either the absolute value or both types of information.

Reducing the biasing effects of relative risk presentation

A number of researchers have recently argued that the biasing effects of presenting relative risk reductions can be reduced or eliminated by giving people both relative and absolute risk information (e.g. Edwards *et al.* 1999, 2001; Muhlhauser and Berger 2000; Schechtman 2002). Edwards *et al.* (1999), for example, recommended that researchers should present results with both absolute and relative risk estimates and not present either in isolation, as this may be misleading or insufficiently helpful for arriving at a decision. Others have suggested that it is important to provide the baseline level of risk as well as the relative risk reduction (e.g. Leung 2002). Thus, in the case of the 'pill scare', women should not only have been told that there was twice the risk of thrombosis with the third generation pill, but that the initial level was only around 15 cases per 100,000 users per annum. My research group therefore recently carried out a number of experiments to assess whether relative risk presentations are as influential if people are provided with the baseline level of risk, and whether the provision of baseline information is more or less helpful than presenting information about both relative and absolute risk reductions concurrently (Natter and Berry, 2004). In these studies, people were given a fictitious scenario in which they were told that Britain would be hit by a severe influenza epidemic and that it was advised that they should be vaccinated. We manipulated the way in which the information about the benefits of vaccination was presented, so that people were either told the absolute or the relative risk reduction, or both, and this information was presented either with or without information about baseline risk of influenza being given. We found that the key factor was presenting people with the baseline information. This led to increased ratings of satisfaction, perceived effectiveness of vaccination and intention to be vaccinated. Providing both the combined relative and absolute presentation formats conveyed no additional benefits over presenting the absolute risk together with the baseline information. The effects held in student and general population samples.

Number needed to treat and odds ratio

A related risk measure that has been advocated by several health researchers and professionals in recent years (e.g. Nuovo *et al.* 2002) is number needed to treat (NNT). The measure is simply the reciprocal of absolute risk reduction. In practice, the measure tells us the number of patients that need to be treated to get the desired effect in one patient. Nuovo *et al.* (2002) argued that reporting NNT provides readers with additional information to help them decide whether or not a particular treatment should be used, and that failure to report it may influence the interpretation of study results. In order to assess the extent of its usage, they examined the frequency of reporting of NNT and absolute risk reduction, in addition to relative risk reduction, in randomized control trials. They found that of the 359 eligible studies, only 8 reported NNT and 10 reported absolute risk reduction. By far the majority reported only relative risk levels. This is despite the fact that use of both NNT and absolute risk reduction are advocated in the current Consolidated Standards of Reporting Trials (CONSORT) guidelines (Begg *et al.* 1996; Altmann *et al.* 2001).

The odds ratio is slightly less transparent in that it is the ratio between the odds of the treatment group and the odds of the control group. An odds ratio of less than 1 means that the odds have decreased, whereas an odds ratio of more than 1 means that they have increased. The measure tends to be used in case control studies, in which the relative risk cannot be estimated. It can also be used in retrospective and cross-sectional studies where the goal is to look at associations rather than differences. In this context, Schechtman (2002) recently argued that it is important that practitioners understand what the different risk measures really express and which ones are most appropriate for particular settings.

Framing effects

In the Halpern *et al.* (1989) study described earlier, it was found that the first presentation format (99,991.7 out of 100,000 will not die) led to significantly lower estimates of risk of death than the second format (0.0083 per cent probability of dying). Similarly, in the Fischoff and MacGregor (1983) study on risk perception, it was found that people's estimates of death rates associated with different diseases varied widely depending on whether they were asked how many people died or survived. These are examples of the classic framing effect. It is now well established that people are more likely to opt for particular treatments if told that there is a 95 per cent chance of survival (i.e. using a positive frame) rather than if they are told that there is a 95 per cent risk of dying (i.e. using a negative frame). McNeil *et al.* (1982), for instance, asked people to imagine that they had lung cancer and to choose between surgery or radiation therapy. Some participants were presented with information about cumulative risk of surviving for varying lengths of time after treatment, whereas others were given the same information framed in terms of dying. They found that framing the information in terms of dying reduced the percentage of participants choosing radiation therapy over surgery from 44 to 18 per cent. The effect was equally strong for physicians as for lay people. Similar results were reported in a more recent study by Gurm and Litaker (2000), who presented patients with one of two videos describing angioplasty and its associated risks. They found that the patients were more likely to opt for treatment when the video framed the procedure as 99 per cent safe, compared with there being a likelihood of complication of 1 in 100.

Positive framing has not only been shown to affect people's treatment preferences, but has also been shown to improve their understanding of the information presented. Armstrong *et al.* (2002) presented risk information using survival or mortality curves (or a combination of both) and found that people who received survival curves were significantly more accurate in answering questions about the information, as well as being significantly more likely to opt for the treatment in question, than people who received mortality curves.

Different types of framing and their effects

Whereas positive framing has generally been found to be more influential than negative framing, other studies have shown that framing information in terms of losses can be more influential than framing the same information in terms of gains. Thus, when encouraging people to undergo some form of health screening, it has been found that telling them about the risks of not being screened (loss framing) leads to a greater uptake of the recommended behaviour than telling them about the benefits from being screened (gain framing). The findings are not entirely consistent in this area, however, and some studies have shown an advantage from using gain framed messages. Rothman and Salovey (1997), for instance, found that people who read a gain-framed brochure about sunscreen use were significantly more likely to request sunscreen and to intend to apply it repeatedly while at the beach, than people who read a loss-framed brochure. Rothman and Salovey suggested that differences in effectiveness of the different forms of framing might result from whether the behaviour that is being promoted is a detection or a prevention behaviour. After reviewing a number of studies, they argued that loss framing is generally more effective in relation to detection behaviours, such as undergoing screening, whereas gain framing is generally more effective in relation to prevention behaviours, such as applying sunscreen or being vaccinated.

Levin *et al.* (1998) distinguished between three different types of framing, these being:

♦ attribute framing; that is, positive as opposed to negative labelling (e.g. 70 per cent fat free or 30 per cent fat content);
♦ goal framing; that is, describing the positive gains that follow from particular activities (such as being vaccinated) as opposed to the negative effect of not taking the action; and
♦ risky choice framing; that is, avoiding unfavourable outcomes (such as injuries or losing money) as opposed to achieving favourable ones (such as winning a competition or a sum of money).

After reviewing a number of studies, Levin *et al.* suggested that there is more consistent evidence for attribute and risky choice framing than for goal framing.

Studies have also shown that a number of factors can moderate the size of framing effects. Maheswaren and Meyers-Levy (1990), for example, found that negatively framed messages were more persuasive than positively framed messages when people showed higher levels of involvement in the situation. Similarly, Cameron and Leventhal (1995) found that framing effects depended on the degree of perceived vulnerability that people felt. More recently, Broemer (2002) found that highly 'ambivalent' participants were more strongly persuaded by positively framed messages, whereas those who were low in ambivalence were more persuaded by negatively framed messages.

Loss aversion

More generally, however, it has been shown that people tend to be more sensitive to potential losses than to potential gains. For example, Kahneman and Tversky (1984) found that people were very reluctant to bet when offered the chance to win $20 if a tossed coin came up heads but lose $10 if it came up tails. A related phenomenon is the 'sunk-cost effect', in which additional resources are expended to justify some previous commitment. Thus people act as though, having made a commitment, they are obliged to 'keep going'. Once funds or other resources have been committed or 'sunk' into a plan, the best way to prevent wasting them is to invest more. Bornstein and Chapman (1995) have explained the effect by arguing that people adopt an 'anti-waste' heuristic. However, others (e.g. Arkes and Blumer 1985) have accounted for it in terms of 'minimizing regret'. As we will see shortly, anticipated regret can have a significant influence on our judgements and decisions.

Omission bias

Other studies have shown that people often opt for inaction rather than action. Ritov and Baron (1990), for instance, carried out an experiment in which people had to decide whether or not to have their child vaccinated against the risk of a particular disease, such as measles. They found that when the vaccine was said to have potentially fatal side-effects, many people chose not to have the child vaccinated, even though the risk of the vaccine causing death was much lower than the risk of death from the disease itself. The parents were particularly concerned about the chances of a negative outcome arising from some positive action that they had taken.

Anticipated regret

Omission bias is related to the phenomenon of anticipated regret, whereby the choices that we make are often affected by the anticipated emotions that they produce. Even choices that seem generally desirable may be avoided if they produce anticipated regret. Thus, in the Ritov and Baron study, it is likely that the parents anticipated higher levels of regret at the possibility of causing their child's death from some action that they had taken, rather than the death simply being caused by their inaction. Similarly, Markman *et al.* (1995) found that decision makers were more likely to feel regret if the negative effects in question were under their control. Richard and Van der Pligt (1991) showed that anticipated regret was an important factor in relation to predicting behavioural intentions. Thus, the intention to practise safer sex may be predicted by the anticipated feeling, 'if I do not use a condom I will feel guilty' (Ogden 2000), where guilt is the anticipated negative emotion.

More generally, Mellors (2000) has proposed that our decisions can be shaped by anticipated emotions, whether they are negative (as in the case of anticipated regret), or positive (as in the case of anticipated pleasure or surprise). Mellors suggested that recourse to anticipated emotions can help to explain why people's judgements sometimes go against subjective utilities. For example, people can show more pleasure at winning £100 than £200, if in the former case they were anticipating winning £10 whereas in the latter they were anticipating winning £1000.

Cumulative risk

Many of the risky events that threaten our lives and health have a low probability of occurring in a particular month or year, but can result in a substantial cumulative risk when viewed over a longer time course. Thus, although the risk of being injured in a car accident each time you drive is rather low (around 1 in 10,000), the chance of being injured at least once during a lifetime of driving is actually about 1 in 3. Similarly, small differences in risk probabilities between different precautionary options in the short term can result in large differences in the long term. Thus, two contraceptives might be 99 per cent and 95 per cent safe when used in a single year. However, when used for five years the 4 per cent difference in effectiveness would increase to 17.7 per cent, and after fifteen years to about 40 per cent (Doyle 1997).

Experimental studies and observations of everyday behaviour have shown that many people have particular difficulty when judging cumulative risks, as opposed to risks of individual events. In principle, telling people the risk from a single exposure to a particular risk source should enable them to infer the risk for a specified number of multiple exposures to that same risk. Unfortunately, evidence suggests otherwise. Shaklee and Fischoff (1990), for example, found that adults generally underestimated the rate at which contraceptive failure accumulates through repeated exposure. Similarly, Linville *et al.* (1993) asked college students to estimate the risks of human immunodeficiency virus (HIV) transmission from a man to a woman as a result of 1, 10 or 100 occurrences of protected sex. They found that for 1 contact the median estimate was 0.10 (a significant overestimation compared with the 'real' level of risk), whereas for 100 contacts the median estimate was only 0.25.

Doyle (1997) asked people to judge the long-term probabilities associated with different periods of exposure to risks that are very small in the short term. He found that people's estimates were particularly inaccurate when they were asked to judge conjunctive (i.e. not becoming pregnant as a result of contraceptive failure) as opposed to disjunctive probabilities (i.e. becoming pregnant at least once as a result of contraceptive failure). On the basis of his findings, he suggested that communicating risks in terms of conjunction framing (which is standard practice in the contraceptive domain) may be causing unnecessary errors in judgement, which could be reduced by switching to a disjunctive perspective.

Weighing up risks and benefits

We have seen in the previous section that people have particular difficulty when interpreting information about cumulative as opposed to individual risks. A further challenge to our cognitive abilities, and thus for risk communicators, is the difficulty that we experience when attempting to weigh up the risks and benefits associated with a particular item or event in order to find an acceptable balance. As Edwards *et al.* (1996) noted, balancing risk and benefit is a very complex exercise. For instance, the risks associated with taking a particular medicine are typically of a totally different nature, form and frequency compared with the benefits. For most patients, there is usually only a single benefit sought from taking a particular medicine, but the potential risks are often multiple.

Edwards *et al.* (1996) suggested that, for an individual patient, a basic risk-benefit (or merit) analysis involves consideration of three main aspects of risk (the seriousness and severity of a reaction, the duration of the adverse effect and the frequency with which it occurs), as well as of three main aspects of benefit (the seriousness of the disease being treated versus the extent of improvement, the time course of the disease versus the reduction in time produced by the treatment and the incidence of disease versus the incidence of improvement due to treatment). Each of these main aspects can be quantified or, at least, graded qualitatively (e.g. as high, medium or low). It can be seen, therefore, that even such a relatively simplified analysis presents a considerable cognitive challenge to many people.

A further complication, as we will see in Chapter 8, is that different people will attach different values to the different dimensions. Thus, risk and benefit are fundamentally evaluative terms. Although in many cases science can inform us about the likely effects of a particular treatment, it cannot inform us about the actual values that people will attach to these effects and the extent to which they see them as being harmful or beneficial. However, our judgements are affected by how much we value the perceived benefits of any particular treatment and how these are weighted against the particular risks. In this context, Veatch (1993) has argued that risk-benefit analysis should be more concerned with the notion of harm rather than risk.

The relationship between risk and benefit

Analytic approaches to decision making have tended to treat risk and benefit as distinct concepts. However, many empirical studies that have asked people to judge risks and benefits have consistently observed an inverse relationship between perceived risk and perceived benefit. Fischoff *et al.* (1978) and Slovic *et al.* (1991b), for instance, found that activities or technologies that were judged to be high in risk tended to be judged low in benefit, and vice versa. Alhakami and Slovic (1994) argued that the inverse relationship is indicative of a confounding of risk and benefit in people's minds, and that this confounding is linked to a person's overall evaluation of the event or item under consideration. More recently, however, Lloyd *et al.* (2001) found evidence for a positive relationship between risk and benefit in relation to informed consent for a surgical procedure. The patients in their study who believed that the operation carried the most risk also believed that it conferred the greatest benefit to health. More worryingly, however, the study found that most patients failed to understand the information about risks and benefits of treatment that they were given prior to surgery. Indeed, some patients' estimates of stroke risk as a result of surgery were actually greater than the perceived benefit of surgery in terms of risk reduction.

Finucane *et al.* (2000) proposed that the commonly observed inverse relationship between risk and benefit occurs because people rely on affect when judging the risk and benefits of specific hazards. They referred to this as the 'affect heuristic'. They suggested that representations of objects and events in people's minds are tagged to varying degrees with affect, and that people consult an 'affective pool' (containing all the positive and negative tags associated with the representation) when making judgements. As is the case with other heuristics, they argued that using readily available affective impressions in this way is typically easier and more effective than weighing up the pros and cons of the individual options. Finucane *et al.* reported two experiments to support their arguments. The first showed that the inverse relationship between risk and benefit was strengthened in a 'time pressure' condition designed to limit the use of analytic thought. The second study confirmed their hypothesis that providing information designed to alter the favourability of one's overall affective evaluation of an item (by providing additional information about its benefits) changes the risk and benefit judgements for that item.

Impact of information about benefits

Some studies have looked specifically at the effects of providing people with information about the benefits of particular treatment options. In a preliminary study (Berry *et al.* 2002b) my research group assessed the effectiveness of telling people about the benefits of a particular medication in order to see whether this offsets the negative effect of providing them with information about the drug's side-effects that we had noted in an earlier study. Interestingly, we found that informing people that a medicine was effective and that their symptoms would disappear in two to three days had no positive effect on perceptions of risk to health or intention to take the medicine. Rather, it seemed as if people expected that a prescribed medicine (in this case a short course antibiotic) would be beneficial. A follow-on study (Bersellini and Berry, 2004), however, showed that the provision of benefit information did lead to reduced perceived risk to health and increased intention to comply when the presented scenario involved a more serious disease (pneumonia as opposed to a throat infection).

Using a different methodology, Vander Stichele *et al.* (2002) investigated the impact of including a benefit message in a patient information leaflet on people's knowledge and on their subjective benefit/risk perception. They found that inclusion of the benefit information resulted in improved knowledge and also influenced people's subjective perception of the benefit/risk ratio. Vander Stichele *et al.* concluded that adding the benefit information helped people to integrate increased knowledge about the treatment into a more balanced benefit/risk assessment.

The role of affect in risk judgements

This chapter, and the vast majority of research in the area of judgement and decision making, have been primarily concerned with how our decisions are governed by our cognitive abilities and limitations. However, as we have seen in the previous section (e.g. in relation to the affect heuristic), emotional or affective factors can also influence our decisions. In particular, a number of researchers have proposed that rather than being epiphenomenal, our emotions and feelings can play a primary role in risk judgements (e.g. Mayer *et al.* 1992; De Steno *et al.* 2000; Hastie 2001; Lowenstein *et al.* 2001; Rottenstreich and Hsee 2001).

Affective states have been shown to influence assessments of the likelihood that certain events will occur. Mayer *et al.* (1992) for example, found that the presence of a positive mood increases frequency estimates for the occurrence of positively valenced events, while the presence of a negative mood increases frequency estimates of negatively valenced events. De Steno *et al.* (2000) noted that the identification of such emotion-specific biases in risk perception has implications for health communication in that they allow for more precise design and targeting of messages aimed at influencing particular health behaviours.

Hastie (2001) noted that one difficulty in relation to looking at the role of affective or emotional factors in decision making is that there seems to be little consensus on the definition of 'emotion'. He therefore defined it as 'reactions to motivationally significant stimuli and situations, including three components: a cognitive appraisal, a significant physiological response, and phenomenal experiences' (p. 671). He added that emotions usually occur in reaction to perception of changes in the current situation that have hedonic or valenced consequences. Hastie pointed out that a key distinction is between emotions that are experienced at the time a decision is made and those that are anticipated or predicted to occur as reactions to consequences.

In a similar vein, Lowenstein *et al.* (2001) proposed a 'risk-as-feelings' hypothesis in which they distinguished between anticipatory and anticipated emotions. They defined anticipatory emotions as immediate visceral reactions (e.g. fear, anxiety and dread) to risk, whereas anticipated emotions are ones that are not 'immediate' but are expected to be experienced in the future. They suggested that although previous research on judgement and decision making has taken some account of anticipated emotions (for instance, in relation to anticipated regret), it has virtually ignored the role of anticipatory emotions. In addition, the authors noted that in contrast to anticipated emotions, anticipatory emotions often result in judgements and decisions which diverge from those resulting from cognitive evaluations.

As is illustrated in Figure 3.1, Lowenstein *et al.*'s hypothesis assumes that 'risky' alternatives are evaluated at a cognitive level, based largely on a consideration of the probability and desirability of their anticipated

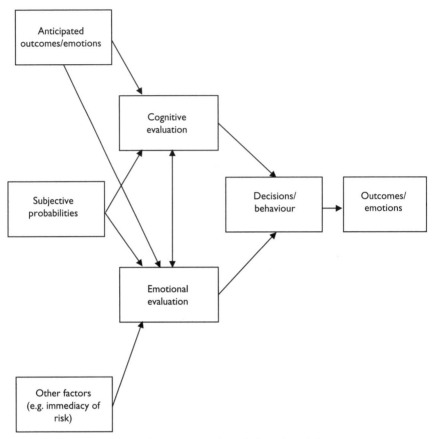

Figure 3.1   Lowenstein *et al.*'s (2001) 'risk-as-feelings' model

consequences. At the same time, however, feeling states respond to these factors in a different way, and also respond to factors (such as immediacy of risk) that have little impact on cognitive evaluations. Because their determinants are different, emotional reactions to risk can diverge from cognitive evaluations. Furthermore, when such divergence occurs, it is the emotional reactions that often drive the resulting behaviour.

Although emotional factors can influence all of us when making decisions, Lowenstein *et al.* proposed that they play a more dominant role in relation to lay people's risk models and judgements than in those of people with expertise in a particular domain, who are more likely to adopt a 'scientific model'. The authors noted that the divergence between the emotional reactions of public and professional appraisals of risk can create a significant dilemma for policy makers, who want to be responsive to public attitudes and opinions but also want to base policy on the best scientific estimates of risk severity.

Expert versus lay models of risk

In general, experts tend to base their risk models and judgements on population-derived statistics of risk probability. However, members of the general
public are often more concerned with their individual level of risk. This can
be illustrated by the patient who asked his doctor, 'What do you mean by
saying that if I have the treatment the risk of stroke is 5 per cent? Surely,
I will not have 5 per cent of a stroke. I will either have a stroke, which is a
100 per cent probability, or I will not, which is 0 per cent'. Thus, people
often hold an 'all or nothing' perspective. Even when they hold a slightly
more sophisticated model, this typically only involves two levels of risk, such
as high and low, or large and small. This suggestion has been encapsulated in
the simplified lay model of risk put forward by Misselbrook (2001) (see also
Davision *et al.* 1991). According to Misselbrook, people are seen as being at
either high or low risk. He gave the example of two neighbours, one who is
overweight, smokes, drinks and takes no exercise; the other who is slim, does
not smoke or drink and jogs daily. The former is judged to be at a high risk
of having a heart attack whereas the other is seen as being at low risk.
However, when the slim, non-smoking jogger has the heart attack it is
necessary to introduce a second element to the model. This is the notion
of fate or bad luck, which results in people using expressions such as 'his
number must have been up'. As can be seen in Figure 3.2, the two elements
(i.e. risk level and the destiny factor) combine to determine the outcome.

Misselbrook proposed that a limitation of scientific models of risk, as
usually held by doctors, is that although they will allow us to predict when
groups of individuals are at risk of a certain illness, they will not necessarily
tell us whether an individual patient will be afflicted. He suggested that
simplified lay models might be more useful in this respect.

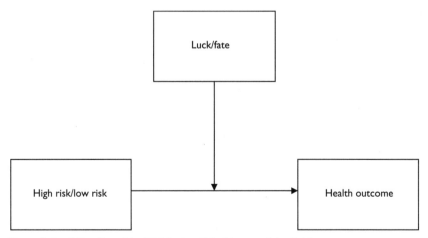

Figure 3.2   Misselbrook's (2001) simplified lay model of risk

The recognition that lay people have 'informed' understanding of risk, by virtue of their everyday experiences of health, illness and related matters, has led to the coinage of the term 'popular epidemiology' to capture this notion of 'unofficial expertise'. Alaszewski and Horlick-Jones (2003) suggested that gaining access to such knowledge is an important prerequisite for effective risk communication, as the specific ways in which language is used to communicate risk information affect the ways in which the information is received, interpreted and used.

Unrealistic optimism

The final way in which risk judgements can be viewed as being 'non-rational' that we will consider in this chapter relates to the phenomenon of 'unrealistic optimism', or 'optimistic bias' as it is also known. A large body of research has shown that people tend to believe that they are less likely to experience negative events and more likely to experience positive events than other people (e.g. Weinstein 1987). Clearly these beliefs may be correct for some people, but they cannot be correct for all people; hence the term 'unrealistic optimism'. Optimistic bias has been observed for many health problems, including the likelihood of developing cancer (e.g. Fontaine and Smith 1995), having a heart attack (e.g. Hoorens and Buunk 1993), suffering from high blood pressure, obesity, stomach ulcers or liver problems (e.g. Harris and Middleton 1994), alcoholism (e.g. Klein 1996), gastritis (e.g. Lek and Bishop 1995), and stroke and food poisoning (e.g. Peterson and De Avila 1995).

It has been argued that the phenomenon of optimistic bias may represent a barrier to effective risk communication. Thus, people exhibiting the bias may not take precautions to protect themselves from a hazard, believing that risk messages are aimed at vulnerable *other* people (see e.g. Weinstein 1989; Shepherd 1999). Most models of health protective behaviour (see Chapter 4) acknowledge the importance of an individual's perception of personal risk status as a precondition for adopting behaviours that reduce risk. In addition, there is empirical evidence to support the suggestion that optimistic bias reduces people's motivation to take precautions (e.g. Weinstein 1982; Burger and Burns 1988; Weinstein and Lyon 1999). Weinstein and Lyon, for example, investigated the intention to conduct home radon testing as a health protective action and found evidence to support the suggestion that optimistic biases about personal risk were acting as barriers to action.

Determinants and explanations of unrealistic optimism

Several determinants of optimistic bias have emerged from research conducted over the past 20 years. Thus, it has been shown that optimistic bias is lower for problems that are perceived to be more likely to occur (e.g. Eiser *et al.* 1993), but higher for hazards where there is a salient stereotype of an 'at risk person'. There is also evidence that the degree to which optimistic bias is exhibited in a risk comparison situation depends on the comparison standard; that is, exactly who people are comparing themselves *with* (e.g. average person, friend etc). Finally, several studies and reviews have shown that bias is higher for problems that people believe they can control (e.g. Weinstein 1987; Hoorens and Buunk 1993; Helweg-Larsen and Shepperd 2001; Klein and Helweg-Larsen 2002), although the strength of the relationship between optimistic bias and perceived control is moderated by variables such as nationality, job status and risk status (Klein and Helweg-Larsen 2002).

There have been two main classes of explanation for optimistic bias, these being cognitive and motivational. Cognitive explanations tend to fall into three main categories. The first draws on the notion of egocentrism (where people have difficulty adopting the perspective of others), the second on the role of experience (in that this makes it easier to imagine being in the risk situation), and the third on stereotypes (in that people compare themselves to an incorrect norm). In contrast, motivational accounts draw on either defensive denial or processes involved in maintaining or enhancing esteem.

Reducing optimistic bias

Given the concern that the phenomenon of optimistic bias may represent a barrier to effective risk communication, there have been several attempts to reduce optimistic bias. These interventions have met with varying degrees of success. Rothman *et al.* (1999), for example, found that viewing a film (designed to emphasize the fact that people similar to them in age, interests and appearance have become HIV positive) increased students' feelings of risk and concern and reduced their optimistic bias. However, Weinstein and Klein (1995) found that asking people to form a mental image (based on five provided risk factors) of someone at high or low risk of having a weight problem increased rather than decreased their level of optimistic bias. Other studies have shown that optimistic bias can be reduced by personal experience of a negative event. For instance, Weinstein *et al.* (2000) investigated the impact of experiencing a tornado on optimistic bias, and found that bias was significantly higher in residents in towns that had been struck by tornados than in those living in comparable 'control' towns. On the basis of this and other studies, it has been suggested that public health campaigns may be more successful if they can change people's perceptions of personal vulnerability. This idea will be returned to in the next chapter, which looks at different models of health behaviours and how they can be used to design interventions to change health behaviours and outcomes.

Understanding and influencing people's health behaviours

CHAPTER 4

What is health?

This chapter starts by considering what is meant by health, as well as the key factors that determine and influence it. It then reviews the main models that have been developed to account for health behaviour and discusses some of their limitations. Finally, it looks at adherence to medicine taking as an example of a health behaviour that affects the vast majority of the population at some point in their lives.

According to the World Health Organization, 'health is a state of complete physical and mental well-being and not merely the absence of disease or infirmity' (Calman 1998: 4). As Calman has noted, several issues follow from this definition. First, health is a relative rather than an absolute term, in that it can always be improved. Second, there are both positive and negative aspects to health; that is, feeling well and ill are parts of the same concept. Finally, health must be considered in a holistic way. Many factors are relevant, including physical, emotional, spiritual, psychological, social and intellectual aspects. The role of many of these factors will be discussed throughout this chapter.

Determinants of health

Many factors contribute to the health of individuals and of populations. Calman (1998) identified the key determinants of health as being:

- genetic factors;
- environmental factors, including the quality of air, water, soil, radiation, and communicable disease;
- lifestyle factors, including diet, smoking, alcohol, exercise and sexual behaviour;

♦ social and economic factors, such as cultural background, employment, income and education; and
♦ relevant health services.

It is likely that in the development of any specific illness several of these factors will be relevant. For example, many diseases and health problems result from a combination of genetic and environmental or lifestyle factors. In addition to this, the level of severity of a particular illness and the likely prognosis may depend on social and economic factors as well as on the availability of relevant health services. As we will see in Chapter 5, these health determinants can be modified by measures to promote or protect health, prevent illness and encourage the active involvement of the public and other key partners. Clearly, effective risk communication can play an important role in relation to this.

Factors influencing the outcome of health care

As well as considering the factors that influence our health, it is also important to consider the factors that determine the outcome of health care. According to Calman (1998), health care is that part of influencing or improving health that requires advice and a service (including prevention and early diagnosis), such treatment or care to be provided by an individual, the community, a voluntary organization or a health care professional. Following on from this, Calman proposed that a health care outcome is the result of one or more episodes of care (including treatment) provided over a period of time, for an individual or community. He identified five factors that affect the outcomes of health care, as follows:

♦ the health status of an individual or community (i.e. in terms of overall fitness or presence of other disease);
♦ the disease itself, including the stage at which it is diagnosed and the likely prognosis;
♦ the treatment, including subsequent rehabilitation;
♦ the skill mix of those providing the care; and
♦ the facilities and resources that are available to provide the care.

These determinants can be modified by factors such as early diagnosis and screening, rehabilitation and the level of involvement of patients, carers and relevant organizations and agencies. Again, effective risk communication is likely to be an important element in this.

Perceptions of health

One of the most important issues in determining health is how we perceive health and illness. Perceptions of health can be one of the most important aids, or barriers, to its improvement. How patients and the public perceive health will determine the extent to which they become involved in decision making about their illnesses and treatments. Our perceptions of health influence, and are influenced by, the health beliefs that we hold. In turn, these health beliefs influence our health behaviours. According to Matarazzo (1984), we can distinguish between health behaviours that have a negative effect, such as smoking, drinking large amounts of alcohol and eating a high-fat diet ('health impairing habits'), and health behaviours that have a positive effect, such as taking regular exercise and undergoing medical check-ups ('health protective behaviours'). This means that health professionals need to influence people's beliefs about both the risks of engaging in health impairing behaviours and the benefits of pursuing health protective behaviours.

Leventhal *et al.* (1985) identified six factors that predict health behaviours, these being social factors (such as learning, modelling and social norms), genetic factors, perceived symptoms, emotional factors (such as fear, anxiety and stress), the beliefs of the patient and the beliefs of health professionals. Clearly, these are related to the factors that influence our health that we identified above. Again, more than one factor is likely to influence any particular health behaviour. The last three will be particularly influenced by the way in which information about the risks and benefits associated with different health behaviours is communicated.

Models of health behaviour

The different aspects of health beliefs have been incorporated into a number of social cognition models of health behaviour. The models have been developed in an attempt to explain, predict and influence health behaviours and outcomes and are based on the assumption that people make behavioural decisions on the basis of their beliefs. In the various models, analyses of the relations between health beliefs and health behaviours have focused on identifying the kinds of belief that should be measured, the rules by which beliefs are integrated or combined in linking them to behaviour, and the conditions under which we should expect strong or weak links between beliefs and behaviour. Five of the most influential social cognition models will be described in this chapter. These are the health belief model, the protection motivation model, the theory of planned behaviour, the transtheoretical model of behaviour change and the self-regulatory model. The first three models are classic examples of expectancy value models. They are based on the assumption that choices between different courses of action are determined by two types of cognition: subjective probabilities that a given action will lead to a set of expected outcomes and evaluation of the outcomes. The individual models delineate the types of beliefs and attitudes that should be used in predicting a particular behaviour, and/or consider the role of additional variables such as subjective norms or perceived behavioural control. The models are clearly rational reasoning models, as it is assumed that people consciously consider the different consequences of the various options before deciding whether or not to engage in particular health behaviours.

The health belief model

This model was originally proposed by Rosenstock (1966) and was further developed by Becker and his colleagues in the 1970s and 1980s. The health belief model was the first analysis of decisions concerning health behaviours that emphasized that 'action' decisions are a function of people's subjective perceptions about a potential health threat and a relevant behaviour. According to the model, perceived threat motivates people to take action, but beliefs about potential behaviours determine the specific plan of attack (Rosenstock 1974; Salovey *et al.* 1998). Threat is operationalized in terms of both perceptions of the severity of a particular health problem and perceptions of the person's susceptibility to that health problem. Thus, effective 'risk communications' will need to emphasize both of these factors in order to influence people's health beliefs. Relevant beliefs concern the perceived benefits of taking appropriate action as well as any perceived barriers to taking that action. Finally, behaviour is driven by internal (e.g. bodily symptoms) or external (e.g. a mass media campaign) cues to action (see Figure 4.1). Later versions of the model have included one or more additional factors, including an individual's general health motivation, behavioural intentions, perceived control and self-efficacy.

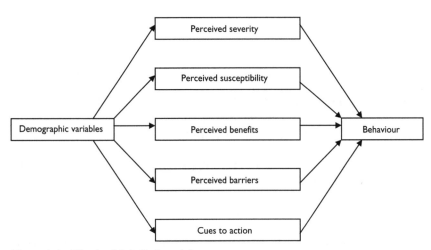

Figure 4.1   The health belief model

Evaluation

The health belief model has been applied to a variety of health behaviours including smoking, dieting, exercise, breast self-examination and condom use (see Sheeran and Abraham 1996 for a review). A number of studies have provided support for the model's predictions. For example, research has shown that eating a healthy diet, having vaccinations, practising safe sex and taking regular exercise are related to an individual's belief that the health concern in question is severe, to their perception of their susceptibility to it, and to their perception that the benefits of action will outweigh any costs that are incurred (see e.g. Becker and Rosenstock 1984; Harrison *et al.* 1992). In addition, studies have provided support for the individual components of the model and for the role of cues to action in predicting health behaviours.

However, other studies have reported conflicting findings and there have been a number of criticisms of the model, including the under-specificity of the interrelationship between the different core beliefs, the absence of a role for emotional factors and the model's static approach to health beliefs. Overall, the evidence suggests that the beliefs specified by the health belief model are prerequisites for preventative health behaviours, but that other cognitions are likely to be involved in prompting such behaviours. In addition, although the model's constructs are frequently significant predictors of behaviour, their effects are usually relatively small (Abraham and Sheeran 1997; Rutter and Quine 2002). A further weakness is that a number of important determinants of health behaviour are not included. For instance, the model does not consider the potentially positive aspects of certain health behaviours (such as the enjoyment of smoking or the thrill of driving fast), or that some behaviours may be engaged in for reasons unrelated to health (e.g. people try to lose weight to look good rather than to be healthier).

The protection motivation model

This second model, which was developed by Rogers (1975), expanded on the health belief model to incorporate additional factors, including the role of fear. According to the protection motivation model, decisions to take action are expected to reflect the degree to which people are motivated to protect themselves. Thus, protection motivation is viewed as 'an intervening variable that has the typical characteristics of a motive: it arouses, sustains, and directs activity' (Rogers 1983: 158). As can be seen in Figure 4.2, the model identifies five components as leading to health behaviours and their preceding intentions. In addition to fear, these are the severity of the health problem and the person's susceptibility to it, the likely effectiveness of any action (i.e. response effectiveness) and the person's personal efficacy in relation to carrying out the action (i.e. self-efficacy). The model describes severity, susceptibility and fear as relating to 'threat appraisal' and response

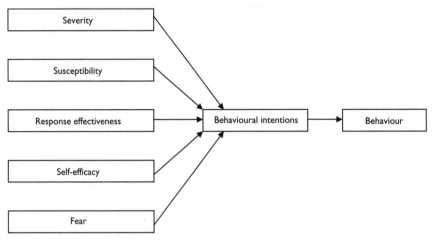

Figure 4.2   The protection motivation model

effectiveness and self-efficacy as relating to 'coping appraisal'. Finally, there are two sources of information (intra-personal and environmental) that influence the five components in eliciting a response (which in turn can be adaptive or maladaptive). According to this model, to be effective, risk messages should not only emphasize severity and susceptibility but should also try to increase people's perceptions of response effectiveness and self-efficacy.

Evaluation

There have been a number of experimental tests of the protection motivation model. In general, studies have shown that self-efficacy and response effectiveness beliefs have been the strongest predictors of behavioural intentions (see e.g. Stanley and Maddux 1986), but there has been little empirical support for an independent effect of severity. In addition, two meta-analyses have been conducted (Floyd *et al.* 2000; Milne *et al.* 2000). Floyd *et al.* reviewed 65 studies covering more than 20 different health behaviours and found that increases in severity, susceptibility, response effectiveness and self-efficacy facilitated adaptive intentions or behaviours. Milne *et al.* also found positive associations between the various components of the model and health behaviours. They concluded that the model is likely to be useful in predicting concurrent behaviour, but of less utility in predicting future behaviour.

The theory of planned behaviour

Although health beliefs go some way towards helping us understand when people will change their health behaviours, it is also recognized that the health belief and protection motivation models have not paid sufficient attention to the role of behavioural intentions and actions. A theory that attempts to link health beliefs directly to behaviour is Azjen's theory of planned behaviour (Azjen 1985, 1988). The model, which builds on the earlier theory of reasoned action (e.g. Azjen and Fishbein 1970), proposes that intentions should be conceptualized as plans of action in pursuit of behavioural goals (Azjen and Madden 1986). Intentions result from three factors or beliefs, these being: the attitude towards a behaviour, subjective norms (including social norms and pressures, such as what other people will think) and perceived behavioural control (which is similar to self-efficacy).

According to the theory, the three factors predict behavioural intentions, which are then linked to behaviour. However, it also acknowledges that perceived behavioural control can have a direct effect on behaviour itself (see Figure 4.3). Thus, in order to influence behavioural intentions and subsequent behaviours, health messages need to address these three factors. Recently, Povey et al. (2000) carried out a study of dieting behaviour to assess whether perceived behavioural control and self-efficacy are separate factors. They found that both factors predicted intention to follow a low-fat diet and eat more fruit and vegetables, but that the stronger predictor of the two was self-efficacy.

Evaluation

Studies have shown that the theory of planned behaviour predicts a broad array of health behaviours, including contraceptive use, breast self-examination, exercise, vitamin taking and sunscreen use. After reviewing the literature, Godin and Kok (1996) reported that components of the theory explained around 40 per cent of the variance in behavioural intentions. More recently, Armitage and Conner (2001) reviewed 185 studies and found that the theory accounted for 39 per cent of variance in intentions and 27 per cent of variance in behaviour. The theory of planned behaviour

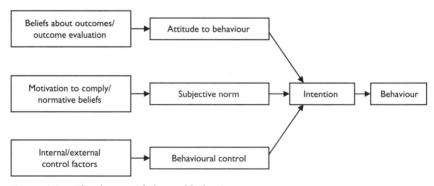

Figure 4.3   The theory of planned behaviour

has received less criticism than the health belief model, but some researchers (e.g. Schwarzer 1992) have argued that a weakness of the theory is that it does not include a temporal element. Thus, the model does not describe either the order of the different beliefs or any direction of causality.

The transtheoretical (or stages of change) model

The models discussed so far can be thought of as 'continuum' models (Weinstein et al. 1998) in that each person is placed along a continuum of action likelihood, according to their perceptions of factors such as risk severity, personal susceptibility, self-efficacy and so on. In contrast, stage models propose that people pass through a number of qualitatively distinct stages in deciding whether or not to adopt a particular health behaviour. Weinstein et al. (1998) identified four defining properties of stage theories of health behaviour: that there must be a classification system to define the stages; that the stages must be ordered; that there should be common barriers to change facing people at the same stage; and that there should be different barriers to change facing people at different stages.

The two main stage theories are the precaution adoption process model (e.g. Weinstein 1988) and the transtheoretical model (e.g. DiClemente and Prochaska 1982). We will look at the latter as it has received more attention and support in the literature. The transtheoretical model separates the process by which a person decides to take action into five stages, with each stage being specified by the person's past behaviour and plans for the future. The model was originally developed to treat addictive disorders, such as drug and alcohol addiction, but has since been applied to many other health behaviours. The five stages are:

1 Precontemplation (where the person initially has no intention to adopt the particular health behaviour).
2 Contemplation (where the person begins to consider behaviour change).
3 Preparation (getting ready to change behaviour in the near future).
4 Action (carrying out the behaviour in question).
5 Maintenance (achieving a steady state and preventing relapse).

These stages are seen as being mutually exclusive.

Evaluation

The model has generated a significant amount of empirical research (for reviews, see Sutton 2000, 2001). It has been successfully applied in several health domains, including weight control, mammography utilization, exercise taking and practising safe sex (Salovey et al. 1988). It should be noted, however, that most support has come from cross-sectional studies (comparing different people in different stages of change) rather than longitudinal studies (examining the same people as they move from stage to stage). Thus, relatively little is known about the causal mechanism that drives progression from one stage to the next. As Weinstein *et al.* (1998) noted, although research has indicated that people at different stages use different techniques and hold different beliefs about behaviour, 'the specific strategies and beliefs that cause them to move from one stage to the next are not currently well identified' (p. 293).

The self-regulatory model

The final model to be considered in this chapter is Leventhal's self-regulatory model (e.g. Leventhal *et al.* 1997). Leventhal's model is actually a model of illness cognitions rather than of health beliefs, but clearly they are related concepts. The self-regulatory model is essentially dynamic and compensatory in nature, in that it describes how a person adjusts to being ill. Leventhal proposed that we take account of five types of information: the identity of the disease; the perceived cause; the time scale of the disease; the likely consequences; and the extent to which the illness can be controlled or cured. The model is divided into three stages: interpretation, coping and appraisal. The first stage covers how people think about the illness and their emotional response to it. In the second stage, individuals start to do something about their illness, either by addressing it (approach coping) or by denying it (avoidance coping). The final stage involves appraisal of the coping strategy.

Evaluation

One problem with the self-regulatory model is that research has suggested that many people do not enter the final appraisal stage, largely because they are only open to one strategy (such as avoidance). More generally, however, a number of studies have produced supportive evidence for the five components of the model and the extent to which they guide behaviour (e.g. Petrie and Weinman 1997; Scharloo and Kaptein 1997). In addition, the model has been shown to be useful in relation to predicting and explaining some compliance behaviours (e.g. Leventhal and Cameron 1987).

Problems with social cognition models

Although the above models can help us to understand present and past health behaviours, and help us to predict future ones, we need to be aware of their limitations. We have already noted a number of specific criticisms that relate to the individual models. In addition, some researchers (e.g. Sutton 2002) have identified more general weaknesses of social cognition models of health behaviour, particularly in relation to using them to effect behaviour change. Neuhauser and Kreps (2003) noted that most of the models tend to emphasize the individual as the decision maker, rather than the influence of the larger social context. As a result, health communication interventions have tended to focus on expert-driven, risk-based information and rational decision making by individuals about discrete behaviour change (Guttman 2000). In a similar vein, Emmons (2000) suggested that improving models of health behaviour will require a greater understanding of how mediating variables of behavioural change are affected by socio-cultural influences.

Of the dominant models, only the theory of planned behaviour includes variables related to the influence of 'important others'. Nevertheless, as Sutton (2002) points out, this model, like the others, offers no guidance in relation to which particular component of the model, nor which key beliefs, to target when developing an intervention. Thus, it is not clear whether risk communications should be aimed at influencing people's attitudes towards the health behaviour in question, their perception of relevant social norms or their beliefs about behavioural control in order to maximise effectiveness. Furthermore, even if key beliefs can be identified, the models do not specify how to go about changing such beliefs. As Eagley and Chaiken (1993) noted, the models provide no formal guidance for choosing arguments to include in messages designed to influence a particular belief. Again, this causes significant problems for people trying to design intervention studies.

The 'intention-behaviour gap'

The largest limitation of the models, however, is the problem known as the 'intention-behaviour gap'. Social cognitive models are based on the assumption that the most immediate and important predictor of behaviour is a person's intention to perform it. Behavioural intentions have been defined as 'instructions that people give themselves to behave in certain ways' (Triandis 1980: 203). They encompass both the direction and the intensity of a decision. However, several meta-analyses have shown that social cognitive models are much better at predicting behavioural intentions than behaviour itself. Sutton (1998), for example, reported that the theory of planned behaviour can explain, on average, 40 to 50 per cent of the variance in intention, compared with only 19 to 38 per cent of the variance in behaviour. Sheeran (2002) carried out a meta-analysis of ten published meta-analyses carried out between 1993 and 2000, covering a total sample size of 82,107, and found that intentions accounted for only 28 per cent of the variance in behaviour.

Sheeran suggested that, in order to understand the intention-behaviour gap, it is useful to decompose the relationship into people with positive intentions who fail to act (which he referred to as 'inclined abstainers') and those who perform the behaviour despite negative intentions to do so (which he termed as 'disinclined actors'). He further argued that the lack of consistency between intention and behaviour is mainly due to inclined abstainers rather than disinclined actors. In other words, it is those people who fail to act on their positive intentions who are mainly responsible for the intention-behaviour gap. Sheeran identified several factors that influence the degree to which intentions affect behaviour, including a person's knowledge, ability, resources and opportunity, as well as a number of personality factors. The type of health behaviour concerned is also a key factor. For example, the relationship has been shown to be much stronger in relation to cancer screening participation than in relation to HIV preventative behaviours. In addition, Sheeran noted that intentions are better predictors of single actions (such as going to the gym this evening) than of broader behavioural goals (such as taking more exercise). Probably the key factor, however, relates to Gollwitzer's (1993, 1999) concept of implementation intentions. Whereas behavioural intentions take the form 'I intend to do X', implementation intentions involve propositions of the form 'I intend to do X in situation Y'. That is, they are much more specific in nature and are tied to a particular context.

In general, studies have shown that people who specify the situation for performing an action are more likely to carry it out than those who do not. For instance, implementation intentions have been found to increase the likelihood of attending for cancer screening as well as the speed of initiating the behaviour (see e.g. Sheeran and Orbell 2000). Positive results have been reported for student, general population and patient samples. Gollwitzer (1999) argued that implementation intentions are effective because the process of specifying where and when one will perform the behaviour means that the environmental cues one has specified elicit the behaviour once these cues are encountered.

Other researchers have addressed the problem of the intention-behaviour gap by expanding on behavioural intentions through the introduction of additional variables, and by looking more at the role of past behaviour. Kanvil and Umeh (2000), for instance, looked at both the health belief model and protection motivation theory in understanding cigarette smoking. They found that only 3 per cent of motivation to smoke could be predicted using health cognition factors. However, the prediction improved to 70 per cent when past behaviour was included in the regression model. Three of the additional variables that have been used to expand on behavioural intentions are self-predictions (i.e. a person's prediction that the intention will be fulfilled), behavioural willingness (i.e. the extent to which the person is willing to perform the behaviour) and perceived need (i.e. the extent to which the person needs to change their behaviour). In practice, it is likely that a subtle combination of factors will determine the relationship between intention and behaviour in a given individual and situation.

Compliance/adherence

One of the most widely researched forms of health behaviour is 'compliance' (or 'adherence' as it is now more often termed), particularly in relation to medicine taking. Compliance can be defined as the extent to which people comply with recommended health regimes. According to Marks *et al.* (2000), compliance in health care takes two main forms: behavioural and medical. The former is concerned with health behaviours such as stopping smoking or taking regular exercise. In contrast, medical compliance can take various forms and covers behaviours such as medicine taking and keeping medical appointments. In recent years, many researchers have argued that we should use the term 'adherence' rather than compliance in order to place a greater emphasis on the patient's role in deciding whether or not to carry out a particular treatment (e.g. Myers and Midence 1998). Leventhal (1993) noted that the conceptual shift from compliance to adherence represents an important first step in moving away from roles emphasizing obedience to instructions and towards models emphasizing the independence or self-regulatory activity of the patient.

Assessing adherence

Studies have shown that the extent of adherence varies depending on the patient population, medical condition and form of treatment, with estimates ranging from 15 per cent to 93 per cent (Myers and Midence 1998). It has been reported that half of the patients with chronic diseases, such as diabetes and hypertension, are non-compliant with medical regimens (Dekker *et al.* 1992). In line with this, several reviews have converged on average estimates of between 30 and 50 per cent adherence across a range of diseases, treatments and patient types. The costs of non-adherence are known to be very high, not only in terms of wasted medicines but also in terms of the additional medical care needed as a result of patients not following prescribed treatments. Non-adherence has been identified as a factor associated with high rates of hospital readmissions.

One reason why estimates of the extent of adherence have been found to vary so much is because it has proved very difficult to assess or measure adherence reliably. Several methods have been used, but each is associated with inherent difficulties. Patients' self-reports and doctors' subjective assessments, for instance, are affected by memory restrictions, bias and expectations. Patients may well want to hide the fact that they have not been taking their medicines or have varied the dosage from that prescribed. Doctors may believe that these patients are much more likely to follow their advice than is in fact the case. Myers and Midence (1998) suggested that patients' reports are more reliable when people say that they have not taken their medicines than when they say that they have. In general, more objective measures, such as pill counts, have shown lower rates of adherence than subjective reports. However, measures such as pill counts only tell us about the number of pills left at any specific point in time. They cannot inform us about whether the 'missing' pills were actually taken or were simply disposed of. Similarly, they do not tell us about particular dosage or the frequency levels at with which the pills were taken. More sophisticated electronic measuring devices are becoming more widely used in order to record when tablets are removed from containers, but again do not provide information about whether patients actually take the medicine in question. Even direct methods of assessing adherence, such as measuring blood or urine levels, or evaluating actual health outcomes, are not fail-safe, given the different rates at which individuals can absorb and metabolize particular drugs.

Determinants of adherence

A large number of studies have attempted to identify specific determinants of adherence in order to develop effective interventions to enhance it. In an early (and now classic) review, Sackett and Haynes (1976) found no clear relationship between race, gender, education, intelligence, marital and occupational status, income or ethnic/cultural background, and compliance. As noted earlier, some studies have shown associations between medical condition and type of treatment and adherence. It has also been reported that the degree of adherence varies with the complexity of drug regime, with simpler regimes being associated with higher levels of compliance (e.g. Raynor 1992). Other researchers have suggested that we need to take account of factors such as the doctor–patient relationship and the patient's health beliefs (e.g. Horne and Weinman 1998; Noble 1998). Horne (1998) noted that people typically hold complex beliefs about their medicines which are likely to affect the degree of adherence. After reviewing the literature, Horne and Weinman (1998) concluded that adherence is clearly multi-factorial, with a large range of determinants, and is best thought of as a state rather than a trait. They argued that we should not talk about individual patients as being either adherent or non-adherent. Rather, we need to achieve a greater understanding of how and why individual patients decide to take some treatments but not others. This involves an assessment and understanding of the particular health beliefs that people hold. In relation to this, Horne and Weinman (1998) reviewed the extent to which current social cognition models of health behaviour provide a complete explanation of specific adherence behaviours, and concluded that no single model appears to be universally valid. In general, the models were better at predicting 'single point' decisions about complying with recommended treatments (e.g. attending for a screening session) rather than at explaining adherence in relation to chronic illnesses.

   Horne (1998) also noted that non-adherence may actually be the intended result of an active decision by the patient, rather than being an accidental or irrational behaviour. In line with this, Donovan and Blake (1992) studied 54 rheumatology patients and found that non-adherence was frequently the result of reasoned decision making. Qualitative analyses of semi-structured interviews revealed that the patients experimented with drug dosages and timing in order to manage the side-effects and perceived effectiveness of the drugs. They made their decisions based on information gleaned from a number of sources, including media, family and friends. In general, the patients wanted much more information about their disease and treatment (particularly the disease aetiology and prognosis and the side-effects of prescribed drugs) in order to make more informed decisions. Donovan and Blake noted that 'the provision of simple information would enable patients to make choices that both fit into their lives and beliefs, and also take into account current medical views about the risks and benefits of drugs' (p. 512). We will return to the 'mismatch' between patient information needs and what they currently receive in Chapters 5 and 6.

Information provision and adherence

Following Ley's classic work in this area (e.g. 1973, 1988) several other researchers have noted the link between provision of information and improved adherence. Raynor (1992), for example, suggested that the provision of information may benefit two types of patient who are non-compliant – namely, those who want to comply but need more information to allow them to do so and those with fears and misconceptions that can be dispelled by providing information. As we will see in Chapter 5, a lively debate has taken place in the literature over the extent to which informing patients about medication side-effects increases the perceived occurrence of side-effects and decreases adherence. In general, it is believed that providing information about particular side-effects does not lead to an increased incidence of those side-effects, although if adverse effects do occur they may be more likely to be attributed to the medicine than to some other cause (e.g. George et al. 1983; Raynor 1992). After reviewing a number of studies, Raynor (1992, 1998) concluded that written information generally has a positive effect on adherence, provided that it is well written and presented in a way that has been shown to be effective, and that the patient is motivated to comply. He noted that additional benefits have also been observed with the provision of tailored or individualized information. In a similar vein, Horne (1998) concluded that improving communication with clear, easily remembered instructions, and tailoring the regime to fit the patient's lifestyle are likely to enhance adherence behaviours. The wider importance of both doctor–patient communication and the provision of clear information will be discussed in the next two chapters.

Communicating information about health and treatment

We saw in the previous chapter that communication and information provision play a key role in determining whether or not people engage in recommended health behaviours, such as adherence to prescribed medication. According to Kreps (2003), communication is a central human process that enables individual and collective adaptation to health risks at many different levels. Thus, 'effective risk communication enables consumers and providers of health care to gather relevant health information that educates them about significant threats to health and helps them identify strategies for avoiding and responding to these threats' (p. 161). Communication can take several different forms, including face-to-face verbal conversations, non-verbal communications, printed messages and those that employ computers and other more advanced techniques. In the next chapter we will look in more detail at the provision of written information, such as patient information leaflets, and in Chapter 7 at the use of graphical and computer-based communication aids. This chapter begins by outlining some general issues involved in communicating health information. It then looks at different models of doctor–patient communication and considers what information patients want to know about their health and potential treatments, and how the provision of such information affects their understanding and behaviour. It focuses particularly on medicine taking, a health behaviour that applies to the vast majority of the population at some stage in their lives. Finally, it looks at health promotion and the difficulties involved in communicating information to the wider population in order to improve public health.

Communicating health information

As Edwards and Hugman (1997) noted, effectively communicating even the simplest and most welcome of messages to a dispersed and disparate audience is a substantial challenge. The problems of communicating copious information on complex scientific or medical matters are even more extraordinary. Communicators may want to achieve any of a number of goals when attempting to communicate with individuals or the wider population, including providing information, instruction or reassurance, influencing opinions and attitudes, and changing behaviour. Edwards and Hugman (1997: 223) identified six core issues that need to be taken into consideration when planning any health communication:

♦ the purpose of the message;
♦ the state of mind of the intended recipients (including their cognitive abilities and emotional state);
♦ the general context or climate in which the message will be received;
♦ the medium of communication to be used;
♦ feedback mechanisms to assess the extent of the effects of the message; and
♦ monitoring and evaluation.

They suggested that clarity concerning these issues is essential if health communications are to have any chance of achieving their desired impact.

The topic of health communication has received increasing attention over the last 10 to 20 years and is now an integral part of medical training in the UK and elsewhere. A significant event in the UK was the publication of the *Patient's Charter*, which informed patients that they had a right 'to be given a clear explanation of any treatment proposed, including any risks and any alternatives, before deciding whether to agree to the treatment' (Department of Health 1992). At a similar time, an international conference on health communication produced what is known as the 'Toronto Consensus Statement on the relationship between communication practices and outcomes' (Simpson *et al.* 1991). The Statement made eight key points:

♦ communication problems in medical practice are important and common;
♦ patient anxiety and dissatisfaction are related to uncertainty and lack of information, explanation and feedback;
♦ doctors often misperceive the amount and type of information that patients want to receive;
♦ improved quality of clinical communication is related to positive health outcomes;
♦ explaining and understanding patient concerns, even when they cannot be resolved, results in a significant fall in anxiety;
♦ greater participation by the patient in the encounter improves satisfaction and compliance, and outcome of the treatment;
♦ the level of psychological distress in patients with serious illness is less when they perceive themselves to have received adequate information;

♦ beneficial clinical communication is routinely possible in clinical practice
and can be achieved during normal clinical encounters, without unduly
prolonging them, provided that the clinician has learned the relevant
techniques.

As Kreps (2002) noted, the quality of interactions between health professionals and 'consumers' has a direct influence on many important health
outcomes. Thus, interpersonal communication may initially be used to
gather relevant information for accurate diagnoses. It is a means of eliciting
relatively personal information from 'consumers' and providing them with
the information needed to select appropriate treatment strategies and to
encourage them to follow the suggested treatment regime. Interpersonal
communication is also needed to gather information that is required to
monitor responses to treatments and to make decisions about refining
care strategies over time. In relation to the domain of cancer, Kreps (2003)
suggested that health communication has great potential to help reduce
cancer risks, incidence, morbidity and mortality while enhancing quality of
life across the continuum of cancer care. Specifically, he argued that effective
communication can encourage cancer prevention, inform cancer detection
and diagnosis, guide cancer treatment, support successful survivorship and
promote the best end-of-life care.

Kreps (2002) also noted that, when looking at interpersonal communication, we need to consider more than the verbal content of the messages that
are exchanged. We also need to take account of factors such as expression
and other non-verbal messages, relational development of empathy, social
support, psychosocial adjustment and situational constraints such as context
and nature of the presenting problem. These can sometimes have a more
significant influence on the recipient's health beliefs and behaviours than
the verbal content of the message, particularly when there is a conflict
between the two. Finally, it is important to consider various demographic
factors, such as age, gender, educational level and culture, as these will also
have a significant effect, especially if there is a mismatch between the two
communicators in relation to these factors.

Doctor–patient communication

According to Ong et al. (1995), the doctor–patient relationship is one of the
most complex of interpersonal relationships. It involves the interaction
between people in non-equal positions, is often non-voluntary, concerns
issues of vital importance, is emotionally laden and requires close co-
operation. Ong et al. suggested that three different purposes of communication between doctors and patients can be distinguished: creating a good
interpersonal relationship; exchange of information; and medical decision
making. We will discuss each of these in turn.

Creating a good interpersonal relationship

A good relationship can be regarded as a prerequisite for optimal medical care. As Roter and Hall (1992) noted, talk is the fundamental instrument by which the doctor–patient relationship is crafted and by which therapeutic goals are achieved. Unfortunately, there is evidence that not all doctor–patient relationships are as positive as many patients would like. Roberts *et al.* (2001), for instance, found that the manner of communication between doctors and patients is still a major cause of patient dissatisfaction, even though it was identified as a cause of non-compliance as early as the 1960s and 1970s. Ley's now classic 1988 review showed that 41 per cent of hospital patients and 28 per cent of general practice patients were dissatisfied with their consultations. Similarly, Richards (1990) reported that most complaints about doctors by patients concerned poor communication rather than competence. Interestingly, the most common complaint was that the doctors did not listen. Unfortunately, there is evidence from more recent studies that the situation has not improved markedly over the past decade or so.

These communication difficulties are a concern, as several studies have shown that successful doctor–patient communication can have an important influence on factors such as patient satisfaction, knowledge and understanding, adherence to treatment and measurable health outcomes. Hall *et al.* (1988), for example, found that adherence was greater among patients whose doctors expressed encouragement, reassurance and support, and was lower when doctors expressed anger, anxiety or other negative emotions. After reviewing the literature, Squier (1990) concluded that there is strong evidence that the affective quality of the doctor–patient relationship is a key determinant of both patient satisfaction and adherence to treatment. In particular, warmth, caring, positive regard, lack of tension and non-verbal expressiveness appear to be the most important elements in establishing and maintaining a good working relationship. More recently, Williams *et al.* (1998) found that the expression of affect during consultations between general practitioners (GPs) and patients was an important factor in relation to patient satisfaction. Specifically, the doctor's friendliness, courteous behaviour, social conversation, encouraging and empathic behaviours, and partnership building all led to greater patient satisfaction. In addition, satisfaction was also associated with higher patient-centredness and empathy during consultations. In terms of actual health outcomes, a review of articles published between 1983 and 1993 (Stewart 1995), showed that quality of communication, both in history taking and discussion of management, was found to have a significant influence on patient health outcomes such as emotional health, symptom resolution, function, physiological measures (blood pressure and blood sugar) and pain control.

Exchange of information

A key element of doctor–patient communication involves the exchange of information between the two parties. From the medical point of view, doctors need to elicit information from patients in order to establish the right diagnosis and treatment plan. From the patients' perspective, two needs have to be met: the need to know and understand and the need to *feel* known and be understood. In order to fulfil both parties' needs, doctors and patients need to alternate between information giving and seeking. As we will see, however, this is not always accomplished.

According to Noble (1998), the manner in which doctors elicit information from patients at the beginning of the consultation can determine the eventual outcome. A number of studies have shown that doctors tend to 'over control' consultations, which impedes the collection of accurate and complete information. Beckman and Frankel (1984), for example, found that patients were interrupted on average 18 seconds after beginning their description of the problem, and that only 23 per cent of them went on to complete their statements. Similarly, Roter and Hall (1989) reported that doctors elicited less than 50 per cent of the medical information available.

In terms of information giving, many patient satisfaction surveys have indicated that, while the majority of patients are largely satisfied with the technical aspects of their care, many are dissatisfied with the amount and quality of information provided (see e.g. National Cancer Alliance 1996; Payne 2002). In line with this, several studies have shown that doctors consistently underestimate the amount of information that patients want (e.g. Daltroy 1993). According to Donovan and Blake (1992), most patients crave more information about their disease and treatments. In particular, they want information about aetiology, symptoms, methods of diagnosis, likely prognoses of disease, nature and effects on symptoms/disease and side-effects of drugs, plus information on any treatment options and self-help techniques available. Noble (1998) noted that many patients lack even the most basic information about their treatments. She also suggested that when illnesses are severe or terminal, doctors are particularly wary about giving patients full information about their illness, its prognosis and the effectiveness of different treatments. However, studies have shown that the majority of seriously and terminally ill patients want to be given such information. Blanchard *et al.* (1988), for instance, reported that 92 per cent of cancer patients wanted to receive all relevant information about their disease, irrespective of whether it was good or bad. We will see shortly that patients particularly want to be given information about any risks that are associated with the various treatment options.

Exchange of information is an integral part of obtaining informed consent from patients, and several researchers have pointed out that doctors' communication skills play an important role in this. Hall (2001), for instance, argued that whatever information ethicists think patients ought to be given about their condition and treatment is of little account if doctors do not have the communication skills to transfer it successfully. He pointed out, however, that obtaining informed consent appeared to be 'little more than a ritual' for many doctors. In line with this, Edwards *et al.* (1998) carried out a comprehensive review of random controlled trials and found that, although many doctors seemed to be aware that patients may not have fully understood what was going on, this did not appear to be a significant concern for them. More generally, Payne (2002) has argued that providing patients with appropriate information is necessary to facilitate their involvement in any medical decision making. She cited a recent editorial in the *British Medical Journal* which proposed that 'patients cannot participate in decision making to the desired extent unless they have the right types of information, given in ways optimal for their own level of understanding' (Fallowfield 2001: 1144).

Medical decision making

The third purpose of communication identified by Ong *et al.* (1995) is medical decision making. As discussed in Chapter 1, the traditional relationship between doctor and patient was paternalistic, whereby doctors made all the decisions and communication was in one direction and was limited. However, during the last two decades, this has been replaced increasingly by patient-centred medicine and shared decision making. Patient-centred medicine stresses the importance of understanding patients' experiences of their illnesses, as well as relevant social and psychological factors. It involves the doctor employing active listening skills to encourage patients to express their agendas, attempting to understand the patient's point of view and expectations, and working with patients to find common ground regarding management. In addition to this, shared decision making also entails the patient's active involvement in medical decision making.

According to Charles *et al.* (1997), shared decision making offers a potential middle choice between two polar extremes: paternalism and informed decision making. The latter mostly limits the doctor's role to one of transferring information, enhancing the patient's ability to engage in autonomous decision making and giving patients the responsibility for treatment choice. As Quill and Brody (1996) noted, in the informed decision making model the doctor can become an impediment to, rather than a resource for, decision making. This has the danger that doctors may regress from refusing to express their recommendations to not valuing them or even formulating them. Their primary role in this model is to cover various options, the odds associated with them and the implications for treatment, to inform patients about their medical options and then to carry out the patient's decisions.

Braddock *et al.* (1999) assessed the nature and completeness of informed decision making in routine office visits of both primary care physicians and surgeons, and found that overall the completeness of informed decision making was low. Indeed, only nine per cent of decisions made met the specified criteria for completeness. Braddock *et al.* concluded that the 'ethical model' of informed decision making is not routinely applied in practice. Several studies have shown, however, that many patients do not want to assume the full decision making control implied by the informed decision making model. Thus, although patients want to be given more information about their illnesses and treatments, many still want the doctor to assume the role of primary decision maker. Sutherland *et al.* (1989), for example, found that whereas the majority of cancer patients in their study felt that they did not receive enough information about their condition, only 23 per cent wanted to have more say in terms of actual decision making. The situation is exacerbated by the fact that many clinicians underestimate patient preferences for more information but overestimate their desire for participation in decision making (see e.g. Strull *et al.* 1984). Studies have shown that patients who are seriously ill are more likely to want doctors to take control of decision making. Similarly, it has been found that elderly people are less likely than their younger counterparts to want to make their own decisions about their health and treatments (Schneider 1998).

In contrast to these two extreme positions, shared decision making involves a two-way exchange of information, whereby both doctor and patient reveal treatment preferences and both agree on the decision to implement. Charles *et al.* (1997) outlined a model of shared decision making that has four main characteristics:

♦ both the patient and doctor are involved;
♦ both parties share information;
♦ both take steps to build consensus about preferred treatment; and
♦ agreement is reached about which treatment to implement.

Charles *et al.* suggested that the doctor has to establish an atmosphere in which patients feel that their views are valued and needed, as both parties have knowledge that is relevant for the consultation. Unfortunately, several studies have shown that many doctors and patients do not fully engage in shared decision making. Stevenson *et al.* (2000), for example, examined 62 recorded GP consultations and interviewed the doctors and patients concerned. They found little evidence that both parties participated in the decision making process, and that there was little foundation on which to build consensus about preferred treatment. The situation may not be as bleak as it seems, however, as in practice many clinical decision making interactions typically reflect some form of hybrid model, with the extent of shared decision making depending on characteristics of both the doctor and the patient, and on the nature of the presenting problem (see e.g. Charles *et al.* 1999).

Factors that affect doctor–patient communication

Edelmann (2000: 111) outlined a number of factors that are likely to influence the nature and effectiveness of doctor–patient interactions in general. These include:

♦ characteristics of the health care provider (particularly gender);
♦ characteristics of the patient (including gender, social class, education, age, attitudes and their desire for information);
♦ differences between the health care provider and patient (in terms of social class and education, attitudes, beliefs and expectations);
♦ situational factors (including patient load, level of acquaintance and nature of the presenting problem).

Clearly, factors such as these will play a significant role in determining the particular decision making model that is adopted in any doctor–patient communication and the likelihood of its successful implementation. Montgomery and Fahey (2001), for instance, argued that the shared model of decision making will be more difficult to achieve if patients' and clinicians' preferences are polarized. They reviewed a number of studies in the areas of cardiovascular disease, cancer, obstetrics and gynaecology, and acute and minor respiratory illness. They found that significant differences between the treatment preferences of patients and health professionals existed in relation to all of the areas examined. However, the direction and magnitude of the differences did not appear to be consistent and varied with the clinical condition of interest.

Improving medical consultations

If the majority of doctor–patient consultations are far from optimal, then we need to consider ways in which they could be improved. Coulter (1999) suggested that the key to successful doctor–patient relationships is to recognize that patients are experts too. The doctor may be well informed about causes of disease, prognosis, treatment options and preventative strategies, but only the patient knows about his or her illness, social circumstances, habits, attitudes to risks, values and preferences. After reviewing the literature to assess the impact of doctor–patient communication on patient health outcomes, Stewart (1995) recommended that when taking the medical history, doctors should ask a wide range of questions, not only about the physical aspects of a patient's problem, but also about his or her fears and concerns, understanding of the problem, expectations of therapy and perceptions of how the problem affects function. Similarly, patients should be encouraged to ask questions and be given clear verbal information supplemented, when possible, by emotional support and written information packages.

In a similar vein, Quirt *et al.* (1997: 19) advocated that in order to facilitate doctor–patient communication and to ensure the adoption of an appropriate model of decision making, doctors should:

♦ ascertain the patient's preferred role in the decision making process;
♦ decide the minimum set of facts that a patient needs to understand in order to make a substantially autonomous decision;
♦ provide the patient with the key information in a form which he or she can understand;
♦ ask explicit questions to ensure that the patient understands the issues and if, after repeated explanation, the patient still does not have a realistic grasp of the key facts, the doctor should elicit the patient's values and, if possible, guide him or her to a decision which is not only consistent with those values, but also consistent with the facts.

Thus, according to Quirt *et al.*, the consultation should start with an attempt to establish the extent to which patients want to take an active role in decision making. Calman *et al.* (1999) similarly suggested that there needs to be a process, logically prior to the discussion of specific options and risks associated with different courses of action, setting out what sort of relationship is actually wanted.

In relation to health communication more generally, Neuhauser and Kreps (2003) recommended the following:

♦ health communication will be more effective if it reaches people on an emotional as well as a rational level;
♦ health communication will be more effective if it relates to people's social or 'life' contexts;
♦ a combination of the effects of interpersonal communication and the reach of mass media communication is needed to change population behaviour;
♦ tailored communications will be more effective than generic messages;
♦ interactive communications will be more effective than one-way communications.

In addition to these general recommendations for improvement, there have been a number of intervention studies aimed specifically at enhancing the communication effectiveness of doctors. Maguire *et al.* (1989), for instance, randomly allocated medical students to either a video-based training group or a conventionally trained group, and found that the quality of diagnostic information obtained from patients by the former group was superior to information usually gained by practising doctors. Furthermore, the skills acquired were still evident some five years after training. However, other studies have suggested that while training can be successful in modifying behaviour patterns (such as increasing the time doctors spend explaining things to and listening to patients), it does not necessarily impact on the outcomes of care (e.g. Putnam *et al.* 1988).

Communication about medicines

A health behaviour that the vast majority of people engage in at some point in their lives is medicine taking. According to McCormick (1996), Osler once remarked that what distinguishes man from the apes is a propensity to take medicines. Thus, many studies of doctor–patient communication and the effectiveness of information provision have focused on this topic. Worryingly, several of these studies have shown that somewhere between 30 and 50 per cent of prescribed medicines are not taken as directed (Misselbrook 2001). Indeed, Beardon et al. (1993) found that 27 per cent of young women did not even cash in their prescriptions. Misselbrook suggested that obtaining medicine and taking medicine relate to separate drives and beliefs, and have separate rules. People may want to be given a prescription in order to legitimize their illness, but they may see taking the medicine as a sign of weakness or they may be concerned about becoming dependent on it.

Despite the fact that a large proportion of doctor–patient consultations involve medicines being prescribed, many studies have shown that patients often lack basic knowledge about their medicines, and that many are dis-satisfied with the nature and amount of information they are given. An early study by Svarstad (1976) found that 50 per cent of patients who were prescribed medication in a neighbourhood health centre did not know how long they were to continue on the medication, 25 per cent did not know the correct dosage and 15 per cent could not report the frequency with which they were to take it. Similarly, Busson and Dunn (1986) reported that half of the respondents in a national survey did not know precisely how, when and with what to take their medicines. There is some evidence that the situation is improving slightly. For example, Lyons et al. (1996) found that 75 per cent of a sample of 100 patients from New Jersey pharmacies indicated that they had been informed by a health professional of the medicine's name, the reason it was prescribed, how often to take it and for how long. However, less than 50 per cent of the sample had been given information about storage conditions, 'over the counter' or prescription medicine interactions, what to do if a dose was missed or how to avoid side-effects. Many of the patients rated these latter types of information to be important and stated that they would have preferred to have been given them.

In addition to patients not being given specific types of information, other studies have shown that there are often misunderstandings between health professionals and patients during medical consultations in relation to medications. Britten et al. (2000), for example, examined misunderstandings associated with prescribing decisions between general practitioners and patients in 35 consultations, and found that misunderstandings occurred in as many as 28 of them. The misunderstandings included relevant patient information being unknown to the doctor, disagreement about the attribution of side-effects, failure of communication about the doctor's decision, and relationship factors. Britten *et al.* claimed that all the mis-understandings were associated with a lack of patient participation in the consultation in terms of voicing expectations and preferences or voicing of responses to doctors' decisions and actions. They were also all associated with potential or actual adverse outcomes such as non-adherence to treat-ment. On the positive side, Donovan and Blake (1992) noted that when patients do understand the information they need to take a medicine safely, error rates can be cut in half and patients suffer fewer adverse effects and have a higher quality of life. There is also a reduction in subsequent visits to the doctor and in hospital admissions or readmissions. Similarly, Miller *et al.* (2003) found that knowledge about details of the treatment regime (when tested eight weeks after treatment onset) was significantly associated with higher levels of adherence in HIV infected patients.

Provision of information about medication side-effects

The provision of information (or lack of it) about medication side-effects seems to be a particular area of difficulty for doctor–patient communications and is often a major source of dissatisfaction for patients. Enlund *et al.* (1991), for instance, found that only 31 per cent of a community sample of 623 patients taking an anti-hypertensive medicine were satisfied with the information that they were given about the medicine's side-effects. It has been proposed that many doctors are reluctant to tell patients about adverse side-effects, fearing that this will increase concern or reduce compliance (e.g. Boyle 1983; Myers 1995). In practice, however, studies have shown that although providing information about side-effects can lead patients to attribute experienced symptoms to particular listed side-effects, it does not increase the likelihood of the adverse effects actually occurring (e.g. Morris and Kanouse 1982; Raynor 1998).

In order to examine the extent of the mismatch between doctors' and patients' views on how much information about side-effects should be given to patients, my research group carried out a series of empirical studies (e.g. Berry *et al.* 1995; Berry *et al.* 1997; Berry *et al.* 1998). In the first of these, we gave a large number of people a hypothetical scenario about visiting the doctor and being prescribed medication, and asked them what questions they would like to ask the doctor about the medicine. On the basis of their responses, we developed a categorization of 16 'question' types, which we subsequently validated by producing explanations for our participants that were based on either the frequently occurring or the less frequently occurring question types. We found that information about medication side-effects was the most sought-after type of information, and that provision of this resulted in highly rated explanations (in terms of satisfaction etc.). After side-effects, people next wanted to know about what the medicine does, any lifestyle changes that they would be required to make while taking it (such as whether they would have to stop drinking alcohol), and how it should be taken (e.g. details of the dose, timing etc.).

In our next study (Berry *et al.* 1997), we asked 18 doctors (including GPs, hospital registrars and consultants) to rate each of the 16 information categories in terms of how important they felt it was for it to be included in an explanation to patients about their medicines. We found that there was almost no relationship between the patients' and the doctors' ratings. The respective rankings (in terms of rated importance) are shown in Table 5.1. The most noticable difference was in terms of the two categories that people in our earlier study thought were most important (namely, information about side-effects and what the medicine actually does). As can be seen, the doctors gave these very low ratings, whereas there was more agreement about the importance of information about lifestyle changes and how to take the medicine.

Similar findings have been reported by Makoul *et al.* (1995) and Mottram and Reed (1997). Makoul *et al.* examined a number of actual consultations between doctors and patients, and also asked doctors to rate the importance of providing particular types of information, as well as how much time they believed that they allocated to this in the consultation. In terms of ratings of importance of the different sorts of information to be communicated, the study found that the doctors gave the highest ratings for providing full instructions for taking the medicine, and the lowest for explaining side-effects. Further questions showed that the doctors rated as most important

Table 5.1 Patients' and doctors' rankings of 16 categories of information about prescribed medication (Berry *et al.* 1997)

Information category	Patients' ranking	Doctors' ranking
Possible side-effects	1	10.5
What the medication does	2	10.5
Lifestyle changes	3	3
Detailed questions about taking medicine	4	2
What is it (drug type etc.)?	5	15
Interaction with medication for long-term use	6	1
What to do if symptoms change/don't change	7	10.5
Probability medication will be effective	8	14
Any alternatives to medication	9	16
Is it known to be effective?	10	13
Does medication treat symptoms or cause?	11	6.5
What if I forget to take or take too much?	12	6.5
Interaction with non-prescription medication	13	4
Risks of not taking the medicine	14	8
Interaction with currently prescribed medication	15	5
How will I know if medication is working?	16	10.5

the tasks that they thought they accomplished most frequently. The results also revealed discrepancies between the doctors' perceptions of information exchange with patients in general and their actual communication with patients. Many GPs overestimated the extent to which they accomplish important communication tasks, especially discussing patients' abilities to follow the suggested treatment plan, finding out what patients think about prescribed medicines and explaining all the risks of any prescribed medicines. In terms of actual communication behaviour, the study showed that, consistent with the importance ratings, the doctors initiated discussion of instructions more often than they did any other topic. Side-effects, precautions and risks were not discussed by doctors or patients in over two thirds of the interactions.

Mottram and Reed (1997) compared the views of GPs, pharmacists and members of the general public regarding the value of pharmacy-generated patient information leaflets, and the different types of information that were included. They found that the pharmacists and members of the public produced very similar ratings of the importance of the different types of information, whereas the GPs differed in their ratings. In particular, the GPs rated the section on medication side-effects as being the least important, whereas pharmacists and lay people rated information on the storage of medicines as being least important.

More recently, Ziegler et al. (2001) estimated that studies have typically shown that between 50 and 90 per cent of patients express a desire for more information about medication side-effects. Ziegler et al. carried out a large-scale questionnaire-based study (with 2300 participants) to determine the amount of information that people want about side-effects. The questionnaire asked people to select one of four choices to reflect their opinion as to the information (about any side-effects, or about serious side-effects) that they would want from the doctor. The four options were:

1 Want to hear about side-effects, no matter how rare.
2 Want to be told if side-effects occurred in 1 in 1000,000 patients.
3 Want to be told if side-effects occurred in 1 in 100 patients.
4 Do not want to be informed about any side-effects.

They found that over three quarters of the sample said that they would want to hear about any side-effects, no matter how rare. Furthermore, over 80 per cent responded that they would want to hear about any serious side-effect, no matter how rare.

Thus, several studies provide consistent evidence for a discrepancy between what patients are routinely informed about medication side-effects and what they would actually like to know. This is a concern as we have already established that improved knowledge is related to better health outcomes. However, even if we accept the position that people want, and should be given, more information about side-effects in order to optimize their care, we are still left with the questions of how much information they should be given and in what particular form. These questions are returned to in Chapters 6 and 8. Before this we will consider particular issues that arise in relation to the communication of information about over the counter (OTC) and herbal and homeopathic medicines. We will then turn our attention to health communications that take place on a much wider scale, and look at the role of health and risk communication in relation to health promotion and public health.

Over the counter medicines

Over the counter (OTC) medicines are becoming an increasingly important part of treatment in the NHS and across the developed world. In 2000, sales of OTC medicines in the UK amounted to £1.6 billion. Such sales are equal to one third of the NHS drugs bill (PAGB 2001). Similarly in the USA in 1999, $82.5 billion was spent on such purchases, with over 100,000 OTC products being available (Sheen and Colin-Jones 2001). In both countries, changes in regulation have resulted in several medicines, which could previously only be obtained with a prescription, becoming available for purchase OTC. Thus, 45 formerly prescription medicines were deregulated by the North American Food and Drugs Administration between 1972 and 1994 (Blenkinsopp and Bradley 1996), and the number has increased since then. One of the key drivers for increased OTC usage is the desire of governments to shift a greater proportion of health care costs to the consumer. In the USA in 1997 it was estimated that $20.6 billion was saved by the OTC retail market (Sheen and Colin-Jones 2001). The number of OTC drugs available varies in different countries, depending on the particular health care system. In some countries, such as Greece, for example, pharmacists can sell antibiotics, whereas this is not permitted in the UK. There are also further restrictions in the UK (but not the USA), in that some OTC medicines can only be sold in registered pharmacies, while others are also available in other retail outlets.

Given that so many medicines are readily available to consumers, it is important that people are provided with comprehensive and easily understandable information about them, so that they can be used effectively. In line with this, the Medicines Control Agency in the UK uses 'information provision' as one of its key criteria in assessing applications for drugs to be transferred from prescription to OTC status. Similarly, the European Commission Directive covering medicines information (EEC 1992), does not distinguish between prescription and OTC medicines; both are required to be accompanied by a comprehensive patient information leaflet, which has to include a list of the drug's side-effects (see Chapter 6). Unfortunately, however, there is a lot of evidence that people either do not read, understand or take account of the information that is provided.

Perceptions, knowledge, and usage of over the counter medicines

A particular concern with OTC medicines is that many consumers assume that the drugs are completely safe, otherwise they would not be so readily available (Clark *et al.* 2001). Vuckovic and Nichter (1997), for example, in a review of the literature on pharmaceutical use in the USA found that OTC medicines were thought to be 'weaker' than prescription medicines and, in some cases, considered 'not to be medicines at all'. Similarly, Bissell *et al.* (2000) reported that many UK consumers view OTC medicines as having far less risks than prescription medicines. In their interviews with consumers, they found that people were much more interested in the benefits of OTC drugs, and rarely considered the risks. OTC medicine use was seen as a routine day-to-day activity.

Possibly because most users assume that OTC medicines are relatively safe, many do not inform their doctors that they are taking such medicines when they attend GP or hospital clinics. Sleath *et al.* (2001), for instance, reported that approximately half of their sample of 414 patients in New Mexico did not inform their doctors about their OTC medicines. Furthermore, only a minority of physicians spontaneously asked patients about such usage. Sleath *et al.* recommended that increased doctor–patient communication should be encouraged so that doctors could detect potential drug interactions, avoid therapeutic duplication problems and gain a fuller picture of patients' health status, and so that the patient could become a collaborative partner in medication management.

In general, studies have shown that, despite the availability of patient information leaflets, people's knowledge of the side-effects and toxicity of OTC medicines is often very poor (e.g. Gilbertson *et al.* 1996). In line with this, Hughes *et al.* (2002) found that only 3 out of 32 people interviewed had actually read the leaflet that accompanied their OTC medicine. The most common reason stated for not having read it was that they had looked at the leaflet on a previous occasion. Similarly, studies have shown that people tend to be less likely to comply with the manufacturer's instructions when storing and taking OTC medicines than when using prescribed medicines, assuming that this will not have any adverse effect on their health (Sinclair *et al.* 2000; Ellen *et al.* 2001; Pates *et al.* 2002).

In 2003, the National Council on Patient Safety and Information commissioned a survey of over 1000 North American adults to determine how well consumers understood essential information about their OTC medicines. They found that more than a third of the sample took more than the recommended dose, believing that this would increase the effectiveness of the product. Only 10 per cent of the sample said that they read the label or leaflet for information about possible side-effects or warnings the first time they bought an OTC product, and 41 per cent believed that non-prescription medicines were too weak to cause any problems. Similarly, Ellen *et al.* (2001) carried out a study with US undergraduate students and found that more than 60 per cent of their OTC drug usage over the prior 30 days was over the recommended dosage. Worryingly, almost 50 per cent of ibuprofen and caffeine tablet users took more than twice the recommended dosage. Some of the misusage of the OTC medicines was intentional (i.e. the users were knowingly aware of their actions) and some was unintentional. The former category included those who used the drugs for their intended purpose and those who used them for 'recreational' purposes. Such misusage is not limited to the USA. Pates *et al.* (2002) surveyed community pharmacies in south Wales and found that 66 per cent of pharmacists were aware of misuse of OTC medicines in their area. The drugs that were most frequently reported to be misused were Kaolin and morphine mixture, Nytol and laxatives. Similarly, Akram (2000) reported that Nytol was the most abused OTC medicine, and that the problem was particularly bad among middle-aged females.

Clearly there is a need for improved communication and information provision for users of OTC medicines, particularly about the risks associated with side-effects and with people not taking them in accordance with the manufacturers' instructions.

Herbal and homeopathic medicines

Herbal and homeopathic medicines are examples of complementary or alternative treatments, as opposed to conventional or orthodox medicines. Other complementary treatments include aromatherapy, acupuncture, manipulative therapy and spiritual healing. Although classed as complementary medicines, it has been noted that herbal products bear more resemblance to standard pharmacotherapeutics than to other complementary treatments (Barratt *et al.* 1999). In its widest usage, the term 'herbal medicines' covers all treatments based on plants and herbs, including some conventional and many homeopathic medicines. Herbal medicine has a much longer history than homeopathic medicine. In fact, the art of herbal medicine is said to be as old as humanity itself. It has been reported that archaeologists have found pollen and flower fragments from several different medicinal plants in Neanderthal tombs in Iraq, dating back some 60,000 years (Tyler 2000). Homeopathic medicines, in contrast, first appeared at the end of the eighteenth century, after being discovered by a young German doctor called Samuel Hahneman. Unlike conventional, and most herbal medicines that treat an illness by using substances that work against a disease and its symptoms, homeopathy uses medicines prepared from a range of natural substances (e.g. plants, insects, minerals) that are 'similar to the illness'. Coffea, for example, the homeopathic medicine based on coffee dilution, is used to treat shaking, agitation and insomnia – effects that are similar to those experienced by coffee drinkers.

The use of homeopathy spread throughout the nineteenth and twentieth centuries so that it is now available in most parts of the world. Thomas *et al.*

(2001), for instance, estimated that 15 per cent of the English population had used OTC homeopathic medicines at some point in their lives. In line with this, the sale of homeopathic medicines in UK pharmacies is said to be increasing by 15–20 per cent per year (Salva and Portell 2001), as it is in the USA. Similarly, the sale of herbal medicines has increased substantially over the past 20 years, after declining somewhat when conventional medicines first became available. Eisenberg *et al.* (1998) reported that the use of self-prescribed herbal medicines within the USA increased from 2.5 per cent in 1990 to 12.1 per cent in 1997, with a total of $5 billion being spent. Similarly, Thomas *et al.* (2001) found that over 30 per cent of a random sample of 5010 adults in England were taking, or had taken, herbal remedies. The Pharmaceutical Society of Great Britain and the Proprietary Association of Great Britain estimated the total sale of herbal products to be between £93 million, for the retail sector, and up to £240 million including direct sales, internet and mail order sales (House of Lords 2000), and the use is just as widespread in many other European countries.

Perceptions and usage of herbal and homeopathic medicines

One of the key reasons for the popularity of herbal and homeopathic medicines is that most people believe that the preparations are natural and therefore completely safe. Reid (2002), for instance, reported that over 70 per cent of homeopathic medicine users surveyed believed that the products could cause no harm. Similarly, the British Medical Association (1990) noted that therapists and patients alike tend to underestimate the risks and overestimate the benefits of herbal and homeopathic medicines. After carrying out an extensive review on herbal medicines, Ernst (2002: 154) summarized the situation with the statement, 'the notion that natural can be equated with harmless is as prevalent as it is misleading'.

In general, most homeopathic medicines are not associated with serious adverse effects, as the amount of the active ingredient tends to be very small. Dantas and Rampes (2000) carried out a systematic review on information regarding adverse effects in homeopathic medicines and found that, although the mean incidence of adverse effects was greater than placebo in controlled clinical trials, the effects were minor and transient. They concluded that homeopathic medicines in high dilution, prescribed by trained professionals, are probably safe and unlikely to provoke severe adverse reactions. However, they noted that it is difficult to draw definitive conclusions due to the poor methodological quality of many of the original reports. In addition, Kayne *et al.* (1999) examined patterns of usage in homeopathic medicine purchasers and found that 40 per cent of respondents were taking the medicines on a relatively long-term basis, despite the fact that most homeopathic medicines are designed for short-term administration. They also noted that 13 per cent of the sample was taking the medicines in combination with prescribed medications.

As far as herbal remedies are concerned, there is now a fair amount of evidence that they can produce adverse drug reactions, which can be serious or occasionally fatal. In many respects the situation is worse than that in relation to prescribed medicines, as information on the effectiveness and degree of safety of herbal medicines is very poorly documented (British Medical Association 1990). In line with this, Tyler (2000) argued that we urgently need more information on the adverse effects of herbs and their interactions with OTC or prescribed drugs. A number of studies are starting to produce such evidence. In the case of herb-drug interactions, for example, after carrying out a systematic review, Izzo and Ernst (2001: 2173) concluded that 'herb drug interactions are a reality and can present a serious risk to human health'.

The situation is exacerbated by the fact that many people who experience adverse reactions and drug interactions do not associate these with the use of the herbal product as they believe that the treatments are harm-free. Furthermore, many users are reluctant to inform their doctors about the use of herbal and homeopathic medicines, and so adverse reactions do not get reported to professionals. Barnes *et al.* (1998) interviewed over 500 herbal medicine users in the UK and found that they were significantly less likely to consult their GP about adverse reactions (even serious ones) for herbal medicine than for conventional OTC medicines. Other studies have shown that between 60 and 70 per cent of patients do not inform doctors about their use of self-prescribed medicines. As a result of this, a number of researchers have recommended that there is a considerable need for improved communication between professionals and the public in relation to herbal medicines, and that it is as important to educate patients about herbal agents as it is to advise them about their prescribed medicines. Worryingly, Tomassoni and Simone (2001) noted that, for many herbal products, there is less information included in the packaging than is needed for their safe use. In line with this, Pinn (2001) recommended that, in order to reduce the risk of adverse reactions and drug interactions, herbal medicines need more standardization and improved labelling for consumers. Similarly, Fugh-Berman (2000) suggested that clinicians should always ask patients about their use of herbal medicines (in a non-judgemental way), as this information is vital for both diagnosis and treatment of their condition, and that they should warn patients about possible relevant drug interactions. Thus, the 'patient should be treated as a partner in watching out for adverse reactions, and should be told about the lack of information on interactions and the need for open communication about the use of herbal medicines' (p. 137).

Health promotion and public health

This chapter has so far been largely concerned with one-to-one communications between individual health professionals, such as doctors, and the consumers of their advice. The goal in many of these interactions is to induce the consumers, or patients, to engage in a particular health behaviour, such as taking a certain medication or having a screening test. Although many of the key issues in risk management and communication are common to both the clinical and public health spheres, the need to communicate with people *en masse* poses additional problems (Calman *et al.* 1999). Thus, when considering how best to communicate risks to the wider population, it is 'essential to move beyond a view of the "public" as a homogeneous mass, or even a collection of individuals with differing views' (Calman *et al.* 1999: 111). Calman *et al.* stressed that communication is therefore more than just a two-way process, as it is also necessary to take account of the interactions between the different stakeholders involved.

Some researchers have argued that the most significant determinant of health is social and economic circumstance, and that the least important is individual health behaviour (e.g. French and Adams 2002). Thus, they recommend that we should be focusing more effort on broader public health education campaigns than on trying to influence behaviour at the individual level, and that health promotion initiatives targeted at large populations are probably the most cost-effective approach to health promotion (Bennett and Murphy 1997). In a similar vein, McCormick (1996) warned that if a doctor advises or treats a patient in ways that are ineffective or harmful, only the patient suffers. However, if a public health policy is ineffective or harmful, whole populations can run the risk of diminished health. In advocating the need for effective health promotion campaigns, he identified what he believed to be the two key problems in relation to public health. The first is that many people currently have unreal expectations of medicine. The second is the existence of medical hubris, which has overvalued the state of our knowledge and has failed to acknowledge the extent of our ignorance.

The recognition that our health depends on our environmental, social and economic circumstances is not a recent one. By the end of the nineteenth century, several studies had identified cause and effect relationships between things people do that could be hazardous and adverse health effects which could result. Linkages were made, for example, between the following:

♦ London smoke and respiratory disease;
♦ sexual behaviour and cervical cancer;
♦ tobacco snuff and cancer of the lining of the nose;
♦ sunlight and skin cancer;
♦ aromatic amines and cancer of the bladder;
♦ contaminated water and cholera.

In order to make these linkages, and to deal with the problems effectively it was, and is, necessary to address the health of the public rather than just of individuals.

Meara (2002: 80) defined risk in public health as 'the probability that a particular adverse event occurs during a stated period of time or results from a particular challenge'. She stressed that it can never be reduced to zero; thus 'safe' is no longer an acceptable term to use. She pointed out, however, that although nothing in life is risk free, some risks are more feared by the public than others. We saw evidence for this in Chapter 2, when we considered the psychometric approach to risk communication (e.g. Slovic 1987) and noted Bennett's (1998) list of risk 'dread factors'.

Promoting good health

Many attempts to improve public health involve health promotion activities. In general, health promotion is any event, process or activity that facilitates the protection or improvement of the health status of individuals, groups, communities or populations (Marks *et al.* 2000). Its main objectives are to prolong life and to improve the quality of life. As Bennett and Murphy (1997) pointed out, health promotion is premised on the understanding that the behaviours in which we engage and the circumstances in which we live impact on our health. Health outcomes that are relevant to health promotion are increasingly recognized to result from a complex interaction between biological, social, environmental and psychological factors. In line with this, the World Health Organization has identified the need for a multiple approach to health promotion which acknowledges the important role that the environment and public policy play in relation to health.

Prior to this, the World Health Organization was largely responsible for shifting the emphasis from thinking about health in terms of the absence of disease and infirmity to emphasizing the positive aspects of health. As early as 1948, it defined health as a 'complete set of physical, mental and social well-being and not merely the absence of disease or infirmity' (World Health Organization 1948). As Kaplan *et al.* (1993) noted, there are two important aspects of this definition that set it apart from previous ones. The first is that, by emphasizing well-being, the World Health Organization abandoned the traditional perspective of defining health in negative terms. The second is that, by recognizing that health status can vary in terms of physical, mental and social well-being, the definition abandoned the exclusive emphasis on physical health that was a characteristic of most earlier definitions.

These changes in emphasis also resulted in a change in focus of public health strategies towards a greater emphasis on health promotion activities. In 1988, the World Health Organization argued that public policy should, as a priority, create environments which foster good health. A subsequent document (World Health Organization 1991) identified both public and economic policy as a means of enhancing the social and physical environment.

Building on this, Tones (1998: 137–8) outlined five basic principles that can be used to summarize the World Health Organization's position:

♦ Health is a positive state; quality of life and not merely quantity is important. It is an essential commodity which people need in order to achieve a socially and economically productive life.
♦ Equity should be the most important concern of health promotion; progress towards the achievement of Health for All will depend on the extent to which inequalities in health within and between nations can be addressed.
♦ Health is not merely an individual responsibility. It is unethical to seek to cajole individuals into adopting healthy habits whilst at the same time failing to take account of the social and structural determinants of health.
♦ Since substantial policy change typically involves a major challenge to existing power bases, health promotion is essentially a political activity. Health promotion must therefore generate political consciousness; it must mobilise communities if it is to take its place as a significant part of the 'New Public Health' movement.
♦ Health is too important to be left to medical professionals and so medical services must be redefined and reoriented.

Tones pointed out that health promotion is the product of health education and healthy public policy. Health education is any intentional activity which is designed to achieve health- or illness-related learning; that is, some relatively permanent change in an individual's capability or disposition. Effective health education can have many significant (positive) effects. Thus, it can produce changes in knowledge and understanding or ways of thinking; it can influence or clarify values; it can bring about some shift in beliefs or attitudes; it can facilitate the learning of new skills; and, importantly, it can lead to desired changes in behaviour or lifestyle (Tones and Tilford 2001). However, it must be emphasized that education alone is unlikely to have a substantial impact on health-related behaviour and on the psychosocial factors underlying it unless it operates within a generally supportive environment.

Health promotion strategies

Countries adopting health promotion as a policy have largely concentrated their efforts on primary prevention activities through the modification of lifestyle factors that account for the greatest number of deaths (e.g. poor diet, smoking and excess intake of alcohol). Two primary strategies that have been used are health education and fiscal and legislative measures, such as compulsory wearing of seatbelts and increased tax on cigarettes. In addition, health promotion can involve strategies aimed at changing the environment in some way in order to protect health; for instance, the introduction of car safety measures such as airbags and roll-bars.

Comparison of the effectiveness of public health strategies that have used education/persuasion with those that have introduced fiscal or legislative changes have shown the latter to be more effective (e.g. Stroebe 2000). However, as Stroebe noted, there are limits to the use of monetary incentives or legal sanctions to influence health behaviours. First, such an approach cannot be applied to all health behaviours. For example, it is not easy to apply legal sanctions or increase taxes if people do not take more physical exercise. Second, the use of such external strategies might actually weaken internal control mechanisms that may have previously had an influence.

In terms of planning specific interventions, Marks *et al.* (2000) identified three main approaches to health promotion: the behavioural change approach, the self-empowerment approach and the collective action approach.

The behavioural change approach

The main objective of this approach is to bring about changes in individual behaviour through changes in people's cognitions. To do this it is usually necessary to increase people's knowledge about the causes of health and illness through the provision of information about health risks and hazards. The approach is based on the assumption that people are rational decision makers and that their cognitions inform their actions. The use of social cognition models, such as the health belief model (e.g. Rosenstock 1966) to plan interventions would be an example of the behavioural change approach. Marks *et al.* (2000) noted that, to date, the approach has had only limited success due to its inability to target important socioeconomic causes of ill health, its focus on the cognitions of individuals and its failure to take sufficient account of individual differences between the intended recipients of health promotion messages.

The self-empowerment approach

The main objective of the self-empowerment approach is to empower individuals to make healthy choices so that they can increase control over their physical, social and internal environments. This is largely done through participatory learning techniques, such as group work, counselling and social skills training. It is based on the assumption that power is a universal resource that can be mobilized by everyone. However, this seems to ignore the fact that there are systematic inequalities that are known to exist with regard to access to material and psychological resources. As with the former approach, the self-empowerment approach has also been criticized for focusing upon the individual as the 'target for change'.

The collective action approach

The main aim of this approach to health promotion is to improve health by addressing the important socioeconomic and environmental determinants of health. Specifically, the key objective is to modify the relevant social, economic and physical structures that generate ill health. In order to achieve this, however, individuals must act collectively to improve their social and physical environments. The approach is therefore based on the assumption that individuals share sufficient interests to allow them to act in the necessary collective way. Clearly, the collective action approach is considerably more political than the other two approaches and, to be effective, can require significant resources.

It should be apparent that communication and information provision play an important role in all three approaches, although the way that they do so will differ. Both the type of information required and the most effective mode of delivery will depend on whether the aim of the planned health promotion campaign is to change individual behaviour, to empower individuals or to address the key socioeconomic and environmental determinants of health.

If one accepts Becker's (1976) proposition that most deaths are, to some extent, self-inflicted, in that they could have been postponed if people had engaged in a healthier lifestyle, then this has important implications for individual decision making and public health policy (Stroebe 2000). At the individual level, the implication is that people are free to decide whether or not they want to engage in particular health-impairing behaviours (such as smoking). The important implication for public health policy then is that it must be ensured that people's choices are well informed ones. Some writers have argued that it is inappropriate for governments to try to influence individual health behaviours by introducing fiscal or legislative changes. Clearly, there are some situations where government interventions are made for the 'public good'. This is particularly the case where individual health-impairing behaviours might place other people at risk (e.g. the need to legislate against drinking and driving). However, if particular health-impairing behaviours only change an individual's health, the situation is less clear-cut. Thus, how strongly should people be encouraged, or forced, to eat low-fat diets or take more physical exercise? These and other ethical questions will be considered in the final chapter of this book. First, Chapter 6 focuses on one particular communication method that has been extensively used to influence individual health behaviours and as part of public health campaigns: written information leaflets, and Chapter 7 looks at other methods of communicating health and risk information, including the use of new technology and the internet.

CHAPTER
6

Patient information leaflets and the provision of written information

Chapter 5 looked at a number of different forms of communication between health professionals and consumers. It was noted that one purpose of such communication is the exchange of information. In recent years an increasingly common way of exchanging information, in one direction at least, has been through the provision of patient information materials. These materials can take a number of different forms including videos, multimedia technology and the internet. Chapter 7 looks at the use of 'new' technology in communicating health information, while this chapter focuses on the provision of written information, particularly patient information leaflets. It begins by looking at some of the effects of providing written information and then assesses the availability and quality of existing patient information leaflets. As Coulter *et al.* (1998) pointed out, patient information leaflets can serve a number of purposes. These include promoting better health and preventing disease, encouraging self-care and reducing inappropriate service use, ensuring the appropriateness of treatment decisions and improving the effectiveness of clinical care. The latter half of this chapter will focus on the provision and effectiveness of information about medicines. After considering the extent of regulations governing the availability of medicine information leaflets in various countries, it looks particularly at guidelines that have been issued by the EC for describing information about the occurrence of medication side-effects. It describes a number of empirical studies that have been carried out to assess the effectiveness and likely impact of the EC's recommendations. Finally, it considers some general issues that arise from these studies in relation to the effective communication of risk information.

Effects of providing written information

We saw in Chapter 5 that providing people with information about their illnesses and treatments can have a positive effect not only on patient satisfaction but also on important health outcomes. Bishop *et al.* (1996), for example, found that people with rheumatoid arthritis who received an information leaflet showed an increase in knowledge about their condition and reported less pain and decreased depression. Similarly, MacFarlane *et al.* (1997) found that issuing a leaflet to patients with respiratory infections reduced their re-consultation rates. Several researchers have argued that providing information in written form is more effective than via spoken communications (e.g. Ley 1988; Ley and Llewellyn 1995; Raynor 1998). Early studies by Ley (1973), for instance, showed that after five minutes patients had forgotten about half of the spoken information given to them in the consultation. Similarly, Wilson *et al.* (1992) found that, after 24 hours, patients could remember only a third of the spoken information given to them by pharmacists. However, there is also evidence that the combination of the two forms of information can be more effective than providing written information alone. Raynor (1998) suggested that the combination of written and spoken information can maximize effectiveness through mechanisms such as repetition, reinforcement and signalling importance. In addition, Morris (1989) pointed out that the strongest beneficial effects are often shown when written information is combined with other educational interventions, including videos, talks and one-to-one communications. Similarly, most researchers and health professionals would agree that, in the majority of situations, written information should ideally be used to supplement and reinforce information obtained from direct contact with health professionals (see e.g. Semple and McGowan 2002). Whether used in isolation or in combination with other methods, however, it is generally acknowledged that a major benefit of leaflets is that they can be referred to by patients when they are away from the stressful environment of the consultation room. This allows patients to 'refresh and review their knowledge at all stages of their condition' (Kenny *et al.* 1998: 473).

Raynor (1998: 86) suggested that written information has the potential to influence health behaviours in at least three different ways, in that it can influence:

♦ patients who want to follow the recommended treatment but need more information to do so;
♦ patients who have fears and misconceptions that need countering;
♦ patients who are dissatisfied with their care.

Thus, written information materials can be aimed at providing specific instructions, influencing beliefs or generally increasing satisfaction. It must be recognized, however, that providing written information will not necessarily have a positive effect on health behaviours and outcomes, particularly if the information is of poor quality. Detrimental effects may occur if people are given conflicting, overly complex, or too much information. Clearly, what would be considered to be the 'right' amount of information will depend on a number of factors including the educational level of the recipients and the health behaviour in question. As far as medication is concerned, the International Medicine Benefit Risk Foundation (International Medical Benefit Risk Foundation 1993) recommended that the minimum information patients should be given should cover the medicine's name and dose, its purpose and benefit, how it should be taken, and special precautions and adverse effects. Similarly, Mottram and Reed (1997) pointed out that patients need to know certain points of information in order to avoid harm and to derive full benefit from their prescriptions. This information includes how to take the drug, how to store it, how it is expected to help, how to recognize problems (such as adverse effects) and what to do about them if they occur. We will take a more detailed look at the content and effectiveness of medicine information leaflets later in this chapter.

How prevalent and how good are existing patient information leaflets?

Over the past decade we have seen a considerable increase in the availability of patient information leaflets that are freely available to the general public. Despite the growth in use of audio, video, computer technology and the internet for providing patient education materials, the humble leaflet remains the most widely used method for conveying health information (Kenny *et al.* 1998: 471). The Arthritis and Rheumatism Council, for example, produced nearly a million and a half leaflets during 1994–5, and numbers have increased since then. This growth in availability is the result of several factors, including increased regulation (e.g. in relation to medicines), more publications from charities and self-help groups, and enhanced public awareness and demand (see also Mossman *et al.* 1999).

In 1993 a survey by the Audit Commission in the UK found several inadequacies in the availability of written information for patients. The Commission made a number of recommendations for improving the situation – specifically that clinical staff and general managers should work together to:

◆ review the written information currently distributed, as well as the distribution mechanisms;
◆ find out what kind of information patients and relatives want to be given;
◆ provide written information about conditions, procedures and postoperative care;
◆ make written information from national organizations available to patients and caregivers;

♦ allocate resources to help fund the production and purchase of written information;
♦ make clear arrangements for distributing written information at the right time.

As Coulter *et al.* (1998) noted, however, greater access is of little use if the quality of the materials that are provided is poor, in terms of either content or presentation. To be effective, a leaflet must be noticed, read, understood, believed and remembered (Kenny *et al.* 1998). Unfortunately, a recent national survey of written information given to patients (Payne *et al.* 2000) showed that 64 per cent of leaflets could be understood by only 40 per cent of the British population. In addition, many of the leaflets did not meet basic guidelines for legibility and readability.

Coulter *et al.* (1998: 16) listed a number of criteria that have been recommended for evaluating the quality of patient information leaflets, including:

♦ accessibility;
♦ acceptability;
♦ readability and comprehensibility;
♦ style and attractiveness of presentation;
♦ accuracy and reliability of content;
♦ coverage and comprehensiveness;
♦ currency and arrangements for editorial review;
♦ references to sources and strength of evidence;
♦ where to find further information;
♦ credibility of authors, publishers, sponsors;
♦ relevance and utility.

They reported a large-scale empirical study which aimed to identify factors which patients consider to be important in assessing the quality and usefulness of information materials. In doing this, they assessed the extent and nature of information materials available for patients for ten common health problems (e.g. back pain, depression, infertility), and also assessed the quality of these materials. In addition, they developed a set of guidelines for producing what they considered to be high-quality materials. The study involved collecting available information from a range of sources (including health authorities, self-help groups, commercial sources and professional organizations) and giving these to 62 patients in ten focus groups, and to 28 health professionals, for discussion and evaluation.

The focus group discussions identified a number of different purposes for which patients reported needing good-quality information materials. These included the need to understand what is wrong with them, to gain a realistic picture of their likely prognosis and to understand the processes and likely outcomes of potential tests and treatments. In addition, the information should aid their participation in self-care, should inform them about available services and sources of help and help them to identify the best health care providers. Finally, the patients reported that provision of high-quality information materials should provide reassurance and help other people to understand their condition (Coulter *et al.* 1998).

Overall, the findings gave cause for concern in relation to both the availability and the quality of information materials. In particular, it was found that most patients did not receive the information about treatment options that they needed to participate in decision making. In addition, the quality of most of the reviewed patient information materials was unsatisfactory. Specifically, many contained inaccurate and outdated information and few provided appropriate information about treatment risks and side-effects. Topics of relevance were often not included and coverage of treatment options was incomplete. Furthermore, technical terms were not explained, uncertainties were either glossed over or ignored and information about the effectiveness of different treatments was often unreliable or missing. Finally, it was noted that few of the materials actively promoted shared decision making (Coulter *et al.* 1998).

Similar findings to this were reported by Meredith *et al.* (1995) who examined 25 leaflets and contrasted the information given with the information wanted by 5361 patients. They reported that much of the information had considerable shortcomings. Specifically, it lacked uniformity in form and content, topics of relevance to patients were limited, terminology was often poor and the patients' experiences were often at variance with what their doctors had told them.

Improving patient information materials

On the basis of discussions by the patient focus groups and with the health professionals, Coulter *et al.* (1998: xi) made the following recommendations in relation to producing information materials:

♦ involve patients throughout the development process;
♦ involve a wide range of clinical experts;
♦ be specific about the purpose of information and the target audience;
♦ consider information needs of minority groups;
♦ review clinical research evidence and use systematic review;
♦ plan how materials can support shared decision making;
♦ consider cost and feasibility when selecting media;
♦ develop a strategy for distribution;
♦ evaluate materials and how they are used;
♦ publicize availability.

In terms of the actual content of the materials, Coulter *et al.* (1998: xi) recommended that developers should:

♦ use patient questions as a starting point;
♦ ensure that common concerns and misconceptions are addressed;
♦ refer to all relevant treatment or management options;
♦ include honest information about risks and benefits;
♦ include quantitative information where possible;
♦ include checklists and questions to ask the doctor, and sources of further information;
♦ use non-alarmist, non-patronizing language in an active voice;
♦ use structured and concise text with good illustrations;
♦ include references and publication date.

These recommendations are in line with those of a number of other researchers and practitioners (e.g. Kitching 1990; Newton *et al.* 1998; Raynor 1998; Wright 1998). In general, there is a consensus of opinion that the extent to which prose is comprehended is determined largely by the complexity of the sentences and the familiarity of the vocabulary. Thus, when producing written information materials, technical terms should be replaced by everyday counterparts, non-essential information should be eliminated, word and sentence length should be reduced, language structures should be simplified and information should be reordered to enhance coherence. Kenny *et al.* (1998) recommended that all new patient information leaflets should declare an objective score of readability using a standard formula. In relation to this, Albert and Chadwick (1992) suggested that leaflets should not exceed a readability age of 12. However, in aiming for simplicity, authors have to be careful that leaflets do not end up becoming overly patronizing.

In addition, as Newton *et al.* (1998) pointed out, to be meaningful the leaflet content must relate to the reader's existing knowledge. One way of doing this is to use appropriate analogies and concrete examples. In terms of design and layout, materials should incorporate clear headings and use of bullet points, incorporate plenty of white space and use a clear font at least 12 point in size. Finally, in order to be believed, the clinical content of a leaflet should be correct, balanced, unbiased and developed independently of commercial interests. Overall, there is now clear advice from a variety of sources on 'how to write a good leaflet' with respect to style, language, layout, print size, readability, diagrams, colour and numeracy. This includes a number of articles and publications that review the evidence for this advice (e.g. Centre for Health Quality Improvement 1997; Kenny *et al.* 1998; Newton *et al.* 1998).

As a general principle, Wright (1998) has suggested that information design needs to be reader-based rather than text-based (see also Schriver 1997). She emphasized that it is essential to carry out a thorough evaluation of any materials that are produced, and that the process must be intimately involved with the development of the materials (rather than a separate process that is tagged on at the end). In a similar vein, Mayberry and Mayberry

(1996) proposed that the scientific evaluation of patient information must include tests of both readability and comprehension, as well as of the long-term effects of the material. Wright (1998) argued that evaluation requires more than just showing the material to a few people and asking them if they like it or find it helpful. One reason is that people may 'like' leaflets that do not actually lead to good understanding or retention. A study by Livingstone et al. (1993), for example, found that 90 per cent of 312 people evaluating a leaflet about cystic fibrosis said that they found it easy to understand but, nevertheless, more than a third gave the wrong answer when asked about the likelihood that they might have the cystic fibrosis gene. Thus, Wright (1998) recommended that performance-based criteria are needed when evaluating materials. In terms of medicine information leaflets, for example, some specific criteria could be that a certain percentage of people (e.g. 70 per cent) can locate relevant dosage information within a specified time (e.g. 20 seconds), that 80 per cent of readers can demonstrate correct understanding for responding to a hypothetical scenario and that, say, 90 per cent of readers can identify the circumstances in which the medicine should be taken. More broadly, Sless (2001) has noted that setting performance benchmarks for written information for patients involves establishing technical, social, physical, aesthetic and usability criteria. Clearly, therefore, such evaluations need to be well planned and rigorously carried out.

Medicine information leaflets

Patient information leaflets are now being produced for a wide range of illnesses and other health matters. The field is most advanced, however, in relation to the development and distribution of medicine information leaflets. Such leaflets (often referred to in Europe as patient package inserts – PPIs) are now routinely provided with the majority of prescribed and OTC medicines in many countries in the western world.

In the USA, the growing availability of patient information leaflets is the result of a federal mandate (the Federal Healthy People Year 2000 plan) which stated that by the year 2000 useful information must be delivered to 75 per cent of patients receiving new prescriptions. The intention is that this will rise to 95 per cent by 2006 (US Department of Health and Human Sciences 1996). Leaflets will be mandatory for selected drugs with particular risks. The Federal Drug Administration (FDA) steering committee recommended that all information provided to the public must be scientifically accurate, unbiased, easily understood and comprehensive enough to be useful to patients (Marwick 1997). The proposed format is shown in Table 6.1. The preferred route for delivering the information has been through computer-generated leaflets from community pharmacies. Unfortunately, a survey commissioned by the FDA (Traynor 2002) found that, although

Table 6.1 Proposed FDA format for medicine information (Marwick 1997)

Medication name (both generic and brand)
Warnings that are relevant to the patient
Indications for use
Contraindications for use
Precautions to ensure proper use of the medicine
Possible adverse effects
Potential for developing tolerance or dependence
Information on proper use/medication administration techniques
Storage instructions
Recommendations for additional discussion with a health care professional
Disclaimer that the information provided is a summary and is not comprehensive
Publisher and date of publication

89 per cent of newly-filled prescriptions came with written information for consumers, much of the information was incomplete and of limited use to patients. Using predetermined criteria, a panel of 16 pharmacy professionals found that 51 per cent or fewer of the leaflets provided adequate information about contraindications to the prescribed drug. In addition, no more than 53 per cent of the leaflets provided sufficient warning of adverse events, and 45 per cent or fewer described important precautions patients should take when using drugs.

In Australia, legislation was introduced in 1993 which required all new medicines to be accompanied by patient information leaflets (referred to as 'consumer medicines information'). Information in the leaflet had to be consistent with the information in the drug's data sheet, although not all of the information in the data sheet had to be included in the leaflet. As in the USA, the preferred route for delivery of information has been through computer-generated leaflets in community pharmacies (Raynor 2001). In order to exert control over the quality of leaflets, guidelines were commissioned for writing and testing them (Dowling 1996; see also Sless 2001). The guidelines specify, for example, that any literate patient should be able to find at least 90 per cent of what he or she is looking for in the leaflet and should be able to understand 90 per cent of what they find. Sless (2001) noted that the guidelines had been used to develop over 800 consumer information leaflets to date, covering most major therapeutic classes of prescription medicine.

The role of the EC

In some European countries, patient information leaflets have been available for some time. This is particularly the case in the Netherlands, Sweden, France and Germany, although the content and method of distribution varies. The general tradition, however, has been to incorporate leaflets as package inserts, rather than to generate them online in community pharmacies. In many cases, the content of the leaflets is fairly technical (Dickinson *et al.* 2001). In an attempt to increase the availability of materials, and to ensure a degree of consistency, the EC issued a Directive in 1992 (92/27/EEC) which required that all medicines supplied to patients should be accompanied by a comprehensive information leaflet which must include a list of all side-effects referred to in the medicine's summary of product characteristics (previously known as a data sheet), in a form that is understandable to the patient. The Directive came fully into effect in Europe in 1999, following a phasing-in period. It was implemented in the UK through the development of a patient pack dispensing system (i.e. the incorporation of patient package inserts).

In 1996 the EC produced a draft guideline on assessing readability (together with a model leaflet) to be used by manufacturers when producing leaflets. The recommended method was based on that used in Australia (Sless and Wiseman 1994) and involved interviews with potential users to ascertain whether they could find specified key information in the leaflet quickly and easily, and whether they could understand and act upon it. It was recommended that the leaflet would be deemed to be satisfactory if more than 80 per cent of consumers could use it successfully according to these two criteria.

Dickinson *et al.* (2001) carried out an empirical study to evaluate the EC's proposals for producing leaflets. They compared people's ability to use two specially constructed leaflets that were based on either the EC model leaflet or on recognized best practice in information design. Their test involved requiring participants to find and understand 15 key pieces of information in each leaflet (e.g. when the medicine should be taken, how it should be stored and what to do if too much is taken). The results showed that performance was worse with the EC model leaflet; the criterion that 80 per cent of readers should be able to locate and understand the requested information was only reached for 3 of the 15 items, compared with 8 for the leaflet that was based on best practice in information design. Subsequent interviews with the participants confirmed many of the difficulties with the EC leaflet, including the fact that many readers did not understand the information that they were given about drug interactions and contraindications for use.

Do people read medicine information leaflets?

In order to assess the extent to which leaflets were being used by consumers following the implementation of the EC Directive, Raynor and Knapp (2000) carried out a study in community pharmacies in Leeds (UK). Patients were recruited as they collected their prescriptions and were telephoned seven days later for a structured interview. The interviews showed that leaflets were not provided with a third of the prescriptions that were collected. Of those that were provided, 17 per cent of the sample reported that they had taken no notice of the leaflet and 26 per cent said that they had not kept it. Only 40 per cent of the sample said that they had read some of the leaflet, and only 20 per cent said that they had read all of it. Finally, only 7 patients out of the sample of 215 reported taking an action as a direct result of reading the leaflet (e.g. returning to the pharmacy or GP). More recently, Hughes *et al.* (2002) found that although the majority of participants in their study had received a medicine information leaflet when purchasing an OTC medicine, only a small number had actually read it. The most common reason given for not reading it was that it was not the first time that they had purchased the medicine. People were more likely to have read the leaflet if the medicine was new to them, or if they had experienced a particular adverse effect. A particularly startling example of patients either not having read, or not having taken notice of, the information provided in a medicine information leaflet was described by Amery (1999). He referred to a report of the British Medicines Control Agency showing that severe oesophageal reactions had occurred in half of the patients taking a medicine called Fosomax. The patient package insert clearly stated that the tablets had to be taken with a full glass of water but, according to the report, many patients had not done so, with disturbing results.

Standardizing information about medication side-effects

In 1998, the EC published a further guideline to standardize the way in which information about the frequency of occurrence of medication side-effects is described in patient information leaflets. The guideline recommended that the frequency of side-effects could be banded into five groups, based on five verbal descriptors, ranging from '*very rare*' to '*very common*', with each term being associated with a specified range of frequencies of occurrence, as shown in Table 6.2. Thus, according to the guideline, a side-effect should be described as being '*common*', for example, if it occurs in between 1 and 10 per cent of people who take the medicine.

Table 6.2 Recommended verbal descriptors and EC 'assigned frequency bands', together with observed mean estimates (Experiment 1, Berry *et al.* 2002)

Verbal descriptor	EC assigned frequency (%)	Mean probability estimate (%)
Very common	>10	65
Common	1–10	45
Uncommon	0.1–1	18
Rare	0.01–0.1	8
Very rare	<0.01	4

Assessing the EC recommendations

Unfortunately, despite advocating in the guideline that patient information leaflets should be subject to user testing (Dickinson *et al.* 2001), the EC did not use such an evidence-based approach in determining the recommended verbal labels. In collaboration with Theo Raynor and Peter Knapp, I therefore carried out a series of experiments to investigate people's interpretation of the recommended descriptors, and to assess how their use impacts on perception of risk and views about medicine taking (Berry *et al.* 2001, 2002a; Berry *et al.* 2003b; see also Berry *et al.* 2003c for an overview).

In our first experiment, 268 students were presented with a simple but realistic scenario about visiting the doctor and being diagnosed as suffering from either a throat or ear infection. They were prescribed a (hypothetical) short-course antibiotic, which was said to be associated with five side-effects. The probability of occurrence of each side-effect was described using one of the five EC recommended descriptors, and participants were asked to estimate the percentage (or frequency) of the population who would experience the side-effect if they took the medicine. The results (see Table 6.2) showed that there was a considerable discrepancy between our participants' interpretations and the corresponding frequencies that had been 'assigned' to the labels by the EC. For example, our students interpreted the term 'common' to mean 45 per cent, on average, whereas the EC attached this label to the frequency band 1–10 per cent.

Our next two experiments used broader participant samples (a total of 232 members of the general population), and each compared two versions of a short explanation about a medication and its side-effects (again presented in the context of a scenario about visiting the doctor and being prescribed some medicine). In one version, people were told that the side-effects occurred in '15 per cent of people who take the medicine'; in the other version they were told that the side-effects were 'very common', the designated EC term for that probability. In one of the experiments, we used a stratified age sample, with equal numbers of participants in each of three different age groups (18–40, 41–60 and 60+) in order to see if the effects held across the age range. Given that people in the oldest age group are much more likely to be taking prescribed medicines than their younger counterparts (see e.g. Cartwright 1990; McElnay and McCallion 1998), we were particularly interested to see whether use of the EC descriptors would result in significantly enhanced estimates of risk in this population. In both experiments we found that people who were told that the side-effects were 'very common' produced significantly higher probability estimates (in both cases this was around 65 per cent) than those given the numerical value. They were also less satisfied with the information, perceived the side-effects to be more severe, the risk to health to be greater and said that they would be less likely to take the medicine. Importantly, the effects held in *all* the age groups tested.

The final experiment in this series examined how 360 members of the general population interpreted two of the other EC recommended terms ('common' and 'rare'). We again found that people given the EC recommended verbal descriptors produced significantly higher probability estimates, were significantly less satisfied with the information, rated side-effect severity and risk to health to be greater and rated intention to comply lower than those in the equivalent numerical conditions. Strikingly, only 7 out of 180 participants who were given a verbal descriptor provided probability estimates that fell within the EC assigned range (i.e. 1–10 per cent for 'common' and 0.01–0.1 per cent for 'rare').

Overall, our results were remarkably consistent across the four experiments in that, in each case, use of the EC descriptors was not only associated with considerable variability in responses but also led to a gross over-estimation of risk. We argued that, taken together, the findings provided a clear message for the producers of patient information leaflets which accompany medicines. Describing side-effect risk using the five frequency bandings and associated terms outlined in the EC guideline is likely to lead to a significant overestimation of the probability that side-effects will occur. This in turn is likely to affect judgements of perceived risk to health and decisions about whether or not to adhere to the prescribed course of treatment. The findings of these experiments were also in line with two earlier studies carried out in the Netherlands and Germany (Pander Maat and Klaasan 1994; Fischer and Jungermann 1996) which also showed that people may not interpret verbal probability labels in the way that is intended by the communicator. Our experiments went further than the earlier studies, however, in that we provided evidence that these interpretational difficulties can, and do, have a negative impact on people's perceptions of risk and intended health behaviours.

A study with real patients

Of course, a potential criticism of the above experiments is that they were carried out with students and members of the general population, rather than with patients reading leaflets about actual medicines they have been prescribed. We therefore carried out a study with patients in a hospital cardiac rehabilitation clinic, a community pharmacy and a GP asthma clinic (Knapp *et al.* 2001). Reassuringly, our findings were in line with those of our earlier experiments, with patients given the verbal descriptors considerably overestimating the risk of side-effects occurring and rating risk to health to be significantly greater. In terms of the cardiac rehabilitation patients, those who were told that the constipation side-effect was 'common' estimated the likelihood of occurrence to be 34 per cent, compared with 8 per cent for those given the actual numerical value (2.5 per cent). Similarly, those who were told that the pancreatitis side-effect was 'rare' estimated the probability to be 18 per cent, compared with 2 per cent for those given the actual numerical value (0.04 per cent).

How do doctors interpret the recommended descriptors?

One could argue that members of the general population and patients overestimate risk because they believe that side-effects occur with much greater frequency than is typically the case with most medicines. If so, then experienced doctors, who should have much better knowledge about typical incidence rates, should interpret the recommended descriptors in a way that is more in line with the associated EC probability ranges. However, a recent study of ours (Berry *et al.*, in press) which tested 56 hospital doctors has shown otherwise. Like our student and general population samples, the doctors also significantly overestimated the probability of side-effects occurring, given each verbal descriptor, although the degree of overestimation was not as great as that shown by the non-medically trained participants. Thus, for example, the doctors produced mean estimates of 25 per cent and 2 per cent for the terms 'common' and 'rare' respectively, compared with 45 per cent and 8 per cent for the student sample. To put these numbers in context, however, it should be remembered that the EC indicated ranges are 1–10 per cent for 'common' and 0.01–0.1 per cent for 'rare'. Another interesting finding was that the doctors showed more consistency in their responses, in that there was less variability in their numerical estimates.

OTC medicines

The hypothetical and real medicine studies described above involved scenarios/situations where the medicines in question had been prescribed by a GP or hospital doctor. However, as we saw in Chapter 5, a substantial and increasing proportion of medicines are bought OTC, both in the UK and throughout the developed world. In line with this extensive usage, the EC guideline does not differentiate between prescription and OTC medicines; in both cases users must be given comprehensive and understandable information about the medicine's side-effects. We also saw in the previous chapter that people believe that OTC medicines are much safer and associated with less side-effects than prescribed medicines (see e.g. Bissell *et al.* 2000; Ellen *et al.* 2001). Thus, it is important that people are provided with the appropriate information in a form that is meaningful to them.

We therefore thought it important to test whether our earlier findings in relation to interpretation of the EC recommended probability labels with prescribed medicines also applied to situations involving OTC medicines. We also evaluated a second aspect of the EC guideline, which concerned actions to take should side-effects be experienced. Clearly, it is important that consumers are not just given information about side-effects and their likelihood, but are also advised what to do if side-effects occur. The EC recommends that, in such a situation, if the consumer needs to seek help urgently then the term 'immediately' should be used. In contrast, if the situation is less urgent, the recommended term is 'as soon as possible'. Unfortunately, as with the advocated probability descriptors, the recommendation was not based on empirical evidence.

We therefore carried out a two-phase study in which 188 members of the general population were given a scenario about visiting their local pharmacy with a stiff neck and purchasing some Ibuprofen (an anti-inflammatory medicine). In the first phase of the study they were told that the patient information leaflet stated that the medicine was associated with a side-effect (stomach discomfort or pain). The probability of occurrence was either said to be '6 per cent' or 'common' (the recommended EC descriptor for that incidence rate). In addition to estimating the probability that they would experience the side-effect, people rated the information on a number of scales including perceived risk to health and intention to take the medicine. In the second phase, they were told that the medicine was also associated with a rarer side-effect (wheezing or unexplained shortness of breath), and if they experienced this effect they should seek medical help either 'immediately' or 'as soon as possible' (depending on experimental condition). They then had to select, from a given set, which action they would take: for example, 'return to pharmacy' or 'go to hospital casualty department'.

The results of the first phase were completely in line with our earlier studies on prescribed medicines. People who were told that the side-effect was 'common' again produced significantly higher probability estimates and also rated risk to health to be significantly higher and intention to take the medicine significantly lower than those in the numerical presentation condition. In terms of the second phase of the study, there was no significant difference in people's interpretation of 'immediately' and 'as soon as possible'. Thus, there is no evidence to support the EC's recommendation that the former term should be used when consumers need to seek medical help urgently and the latter when the need is less urgent. Again, the EC appears to have been premature in recommending the use of particular terms or phrases, without assessing how people actually interpret their meaning.

Did the EC simply choose the wrong labels?

One conclusion from our experiments is that verbal descriptors should not be used to describe the frequency of occurrence of medication side-effects. However, it could be argued that the use of verbal labels is not necessarily problematic *per se*, but that the EC have simply attached the wrong verbal labels to the specified probability ranges. Indeed, as outlined in Chapter 2, Calman (1996) advocated a different set of verbal labels ('high', 'moderate', 'low', 'very low', 'minimal', and 'negligible') to describe the risk of adverse events such as the occurrence of medication side-effects, when he was Chief Medical Officer in the UK. For example, he recommended that the term

Table 6.3 Mean probability estimates for Calman's (1996) six frequency descriptors, together with the designated frequency bands

Frequency label	Designated band (%)	Mean probability estimate (%)
High	>1	60.5
Moderate	0.1–1	34.4
Low	0.01–0.1	17.2
Very Low	0.001–0.01	10.7
Minimal	0.0001–0.001	9.7
Negligible	<0.0001	8.5

'high risk' should be used for probabilities in the range to which the EC has assigned the term 'common', and 'low risk' for the probability range which the EC has linked to 'rare'. Again, however, the recommendations were not based on empirical evidence, and a recent study by our research group has shown a significant divergence between Calman's recommendations and people's actual interpretations (see Table 6.3). We used a very similar methodology to that used in our earlier study with the EC descriptors (Berry *et al.* 2002a), with participants being required to estimate the probability of particular side-effects occurring given each of the six Calman descriptors. Again, we found that people significantly overestimated the risk of side-effects occurring given each descriptor. The findings were replicated in a second study (Berry *et al.*, in press) in which we compared estimates for a group of university students and a group of hospital doctors. Both groups significantly overestimated the probability of side-effects occurring, given each descriptor, although (as with the EC descriptors) the degree of over-estimation, and the amount of variability in estimates, was not as high for the doctors. In addition, we found that both groups had difficulty distinguishing between the meaning of the three lowest frequency descriptors ('very low', 'minimal' and 'negligible').

So what information should be provided and in what form?

Clearly, if people do considerably overestimate the risk of side-effects occurring when they interpret recommended verbal descriptors, this is a serious concern. Our studies have shown that this misinterpretation affects people's perception of risk to health and intention to take the medicine in question. Thus, use of the descriptors could have a negative effect on health behaviours, such as adherence, and subsequent health outcomes. However, we saw in Chapter 3 that many people also have considerable difficulty interpreting numerical probability information, particularly when presented as percentages. Some researchers have proposed that there may be a benefit from presenting information in both numerical and verbal form, building on the advantages of each (e.g. Wallsten *et al.* 1993), or from using graphical forms of presentation (e.g. Lipkus and Hollands 1999; see Chapter 7). One difficulty with these proposals is that many medicines are associated with a large number of side-effects. Thus, providing information in both numerical and verbal form, or incorporating graphical displays, will significantly lengthen the content of leaflets, and may result in greater confusion.

Despite the fact that empirical studies have provided evidence that the majority of people do want to be told about all side-effects (e.g. Ziegler *et al.* 2001), given the desire to reduce information overload it seems likely that a more practical suggestion would be to inform them only about more frequent or more severe side-effects. This information would need to be integrated with other key information that should be provided about the medicine (e.g. what the drug does, how to store and use it appropriately and the conditions under which it should *not* be taken). In addition, it is important that there is consistency between the content of patient information leaflets for different brands of generically identical drugs, which is not always the case at present. Bjerrum and Fogel (2003) carried out a study in Danish pharmacies and found that different brands of the same generic product included leaflets with substantial inconsistencies, particularly in relation to information about indications for drug use, adverse effects, drug interactions and precautions. This often resulted in confusion and patients having to return to the pharmacy.

It has also been argued that it is important to include information about a medicine's benefits in information leaflets. Amery (1999) pointed out that the current European leaflet format does not allow for a discussion of the treatment's benefits, which results in an unbalanced focus on side-effects. Thus, with the present emphasis on tolerability and safety, the patient may be exposed to a 'relatively negative information overload' (Amery 1999: 122). Amery recommended that if patients are to make a well balanced benefit-risk assessment and obtain maximum benefit from a medicine the leaflet should include information about the expected benefit, its likelihood and the expected time course of the effect. This information needs to be integrated with information about the disease and how the medicine is expected to affect it, as well as the side-effects and interactions that could occur, and measures to avoid these.

Consideration also needs to be given to the order in which the information is presented as this can impact on how well it is processed and remembered (e.g. Berry *et al.* 1998). For example, we found that in order to be remembered, information about drug administration (e.g. details of dosage and how to take the medicine) had to be described at the *start* of the explanation, whereas information about side-effects was remembered irrespective of its relative position in the text. It is likely that the 'order effect' is related to the perceived importance of the information. Subjective ratings showed that information about side-effects was rated as being much more important than information about drug administration. In line with this, Bergus *et al.* (2002) found that when patients evaluate low-risk medical interventions they form less favourable impressions of the treatment and are less likely to consent to treatment when they learn about the risks after the benefits. However, order effects were not observed with high-risk treatments.

Furthermore, designers also need to consider whether the information needs of first-time users will differ markedly from those of people who are collecting repeat prescriptions, many of whom may have been taking a particular medicine for several years. In the latter case, patients may be even more reluctant to read leaflets, as they assume that they already know the necessary information (e.g. Hughes *et al.* 2002). This is clearly problematic when new information about a drug becomes available – for example, about an important adverse effect or contraindication.

In addition to these practical issues, there are many significant and more wide-ranging issues that relate to the questions of what information should be provided and in what form. For example, is standardization necessarily a good thing, what is the appropriate balance of information about risks and benefits, how can information be made meaningful for a particular individual and should leaflets be aimed at getting patients to make informed decisions (even if this means not taking the medicine) or to take their medicines as directed? These and other issues will be addressed in the final chapter of this book. First, Chapter 7 looks at a number of other ways of presenting information about risk to people, including the use of graphics, specially designed risk scales and new technology.

Other risk scales and tools for aiding understanding of health-related information

We saw in Chapters 3 and 6 that people have difficulty interpreting verbal descriptors, such as those recommended by the EC and Calman. We also saw in Chapter 3 that many of us have problems when interpreting numerical probability information. Difficulties such as these have resulted in researchers suggesting a number of other ways of presenting risk information. This chapter begins by looking at some of the specific 'risk scales' that have been devised in an attempt to aid people's understanding. It then considers the use of more general graphical presentation methods. Following this, it assesses the use of new technology for presenting risk and health-related information. As part of this, it looks at a number of computerized decision aids that have been produced in recent years. Finally, it considers the advantages and disadvantages of the internet for presenting risk and health information.

Risk ladders and scales

According to Mohanna and Chambers (2001), a good risk scale should enable risks to be compared and described, and will increase people's understanding about the risks that they are facing. In the area of health, the use of risk scales should lead to decision making that patients and health professionals feel comfortable with, and preferably should increase the likelihood of a positive health outcome. A number of different scales have been specifically developed for presenting risk information over the past ten years or so. We will look at five of them.

Risk ladders

Risk ladders have been used most extensively to convey information about environmental hazards, although some have been modified for use in the arca of health. Typically, risk ladders display a range of risks of different magnitudes, with higher risks being presented higher up the ladder (see Table 7.1). In order to aid understanding, the risk of primary interest is compared with other more familiar risks (such as the risk of being in a road accident or being murdered). The idea is that, at a glance, one should be able to get a feel for the relative size of the risk in question. In an experimental study, Sandman *et al.* (1994) presented people with hypothetical test results of radon and asbestos in homes, on risk ladders in several different formats. The formats varied in terms of whether a comparison item (e.g. smoking) was included, and whether the risk was high or low on the ladder. They found that adding a comparison item made people feel that the information was more helpful, but it did *not* affect their perceptions of threat. However, such perceptions *were* influenced by location of the risk on the ladder, with more perceived threat being associated with the higher of the two positions on the ladder. According to Lipkus and Hollands (1999), risk ladders can help people to 'anchor' a risk to upper- and lower-bound reference points. However, they are less useful for informing people about absolute levels of risk. In addition, their effectiveness depends on people's knowledge about the particular comparison items that are displayed on the scales.

The Paling Perspective scale

This scale, which was developed in the mid-1990s, allows users to place the risks of particular events in order along a logarithmic scale (Paling 1997). In essence, it can be thought of as a type of 'horizontal risk ladder'. The scale runs from 1 in 1 trillion (−6), through 1 in 1 million (0) to 1 in 1 (+6). According to Mohanna and Chambers (2001), it is particularly useful for presenting information about irreversible, as opposed to reversible, risks. As with other types of risk ladder, some people have placed comparison items on the scale, such as the risk of being murdered or killed in a road accident, in order to help people understand the relative magnitude of the primary risk in question. The problem with this (which is also shared with some

Table 7.1 Example of a simplified risk ladder

Cause of death	Risk of an individual dying in one year
Smoking 10 cigarettes a day	1 in 200
All natural causes	1 in 850
Influenza	1 in 5000
Road accident	1 in 8000
Leukemia	1 in 12,500
Murder	1 in 100,000
Hit by lightning	1 in 10 million

other scales) is that people differ in their beliefs about the likelihood of such events, and these biases can then affect their interpretation of the particular health risks in question. Thus, if people think that the risk of being killed in a road accident is considerably lower than it actually is, then this means that they may also underestimate the level of risk associated with the primary event under consideration.

Lee and Mehta (2003) recently evaluated a visual risk communication tool based on the Paling scale, to determine how use of the tool affected knowledge and perception of blood transfusion risk. They compared the Paling version with a text-based format, and found that both resulted in increased knowledge of risk and in decreased perceptions of dread and severity. However, there was no difference between the effectiveness of the Paling and the text-based versions. The Paling scale can be downloaded from the internet at www.healthcarespeaker.com.

The Community Risk scale

Calman and Royston (1997) suggested that, as we are all interested in what risk means for us, our families and our communities, a risk scale based on the size of different 'communities', such as villages, towns and cities, might aid people's understanding. When using the scale, different risk magnitudes are anchored via the community cluster classification. Thus, the occurrence of a particularly high risk could be described as the likelihood of 'one adverse event occurring per family', whereas a lower risk might be described as 'one adverse event per city' and a very small risk as 'one adverse event per country'. A simplified version of the scale is shown in Table 7.2. According to Calman and Royston, the classification is useful as it helps people to think about risk magnitude in terms that they can easily understand. However, although use of the scale might help us to understand the relative sizes of different risks, it can lead to problems when interpreting the absolute risk involved. For example, does it really help us to understand the risk of being

Table 7.2 Simplified version of Calman and Royston's (1997) Community Risk scale

Risk Magnitude	Expect about one adverse event per:	Example: deaths in Britain from:
1 in 1	person	
1 in 10	family	
1 in 100	street	any cause
1 in 1000	village	any cause, age 40
1 in 10,000	small town	road accident
1 in 100,000	large town	murder
1 in 10 million	country	lightning

killed by a lightning strike if we are told that it is likely to happen to about one person per country? People are likely to differ very much in terms of their judgements of how many people live in the average country.

The Lottery scale

Barclay *et al.* (1998) suggested that, given the popularity of the National Lottery in the UK, many people (with a broad range of backgrounds and educational levels) would have experience of buying Lottery tickets and/or of watching the weekly draw on TV. They therefore suggested that a Lottery-based scale might be an effective way of conveying risk information, as many people would have a good understanding of the risk of the selected comparison items (i.e. particular outcomes in the Lottery draw). Based on the figures supplied by the Lottery organizers, Barclay *et al.* designed a near-logarithmic scale showing the probability of matching a number of balls for a £5 stake. For example, a three-ball prize (£10) corresponds to a risk of between 1 in 10 and 1 in 100 (see Table 7.3). They suggested that many people might be expected to have knowledge of how likely these winning events would be, which would enable them to make effective risk comparisons.

Evaluating the Lottery scale

In an attempt to find empirical support for Barclay *et al.*'s suggestion, we carried out two studies to assess the scale's utility. In the first, we asked 132 members of the general population to estimate the probability, given a £5 stake, of their having three, four, five or six numbers match the winning Lottery numbers. Half of the sample were regular Lottery players in that they bought Lottery tickets every, or nearly every, week. Participants indicated their judgements by selecting one of the six verbal descriptors from Calman's scale, and by selecting one of six given numerical frequency bands. We found that people were very poor at selecting the correct probabilities, when presented in either verbal or numerical format. This was particularly the case for the three- and four-ball matches (i.e. the higher probability events), with fewer than 5 per cent of participants providing

Table 7.3 Simplified version of Barclay *et al.*'s Lottery scale

Number of balls	Probability	Verbal scale
3	1:11	High
4	1:206	Moderate
5	1:11,098	Very low
6	1:2,796,763	Negligible

correct responses. The majority of participants greatly underestimated the probabilities, believing that their chances of winning were far less than they were in practice. Thus, indicating that a particular event has the same likelihood as a three-ball win on the Lottery may well lead people to underestimate the likelihood of that risk. Interestingly, there was no difference at all between the responses of those who were regular Lottery players and those who were not.

In the second study we looked more directly at using the Lottery scale as a means of communicating the probability of medication side-effects (compared with more traditional verbal and numerical forms of presentation). We found that people were less satisfied with the Lottery version (e.g. the risk of side-effects is the same as the likelihood of a three-ball win) than with the verbal (e.g. the risk of side-effects is 'high') and numerical (e.g. the risk of side-effects is '9 per cent, i.e. 1 in 11') formats. In addition, all three formats led to significant overestimations of the probability of side-effects occurring (particularly for the higher frequency of the two probability outcomes that was used). However, probability estimates and judgements of risk to health were significantly higher for the verbal condition than for the Lottery and numerical conditions. The verbal condition also led to significantly lower ratings of intention to take the medicine. So, although people were not accurate when judging the probability of different Lottery outcomes, and were less satisfied when the Lottery scale was used to describe the probability of medication side-effects, use of the scale led to lower ratings of risk and higher ratings of compliance than the verbal descriptors.

The Magnifier scale

It has been noted by several researchers that graphical methods of presentation can be particularly effective for conveying information about low probability risks (e.g. Kaplan *et al.* 1985). Building on this, Woloshin *et al.* (2000) developed a risk scale that was specifically aimed at helping people quantify small probabilities. Their Magnifier scale shows a range of magnitudes from 0 to 100 per cent. The range from 0 to 1 per cent is magnified so that low probabilities (e.g. 0.01 per cent) can be meaningfully portrayed (see Figure 7.1). Woloshin *et al.* carried out an empirical study to evaluate the scale's performance for events varying in probability, and compared its validity, reliability and usability with those of three benchmark scales (a linear word scale, a '1 in X scale' and a linear numerical scale similar to the Magnifier scale but without the magnification). Participants assessed the likelihood of six 'familiar' events (e.g. dying from any cause, sustaining a minor injury in a car crash, giving birth to sextuplets) on the four different scales. The results showed that the Magnifier and the two linear scales outperformed the '1 in X' scale on all criteria. The Magnifier scale was rated as easy to use and was felt to be a 'very good' or 'good' indicator of feelings about chance. It was seen as particularly beneficial for facilitating expression

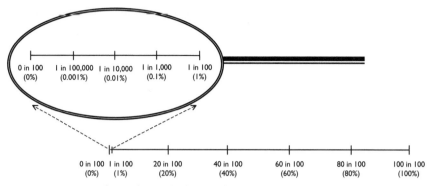

Figure 7.1   Magnifier scale (Woloshin *et al.* 2000)

of low probability judgements. Woloshin *et al.* concluded that although the Magnifier and linear numerical scales were similar in validity, reliability and usability, only the Magnifier scale made it possible to elicit perceptions in the low probability range (i.e. less than 1 per cent).

Generic visual display formats

According to Cleveland and McGill (1984), the primary purpose of a graphical display is not to convey numerical information. Rather, the 'power of a graph is its ability to enable one to take in the quantitative information, organise it, and see patterns and structure not readily revealed by other means of studying the data' (p. 535). Graphs and other visual displays can be used to communicate several different aspects of risk information, such as risk magnitude, degree of uncertainty or variability, cumulative risk, comparisons between two or more risks and interactions between different risk factors. A number of researchers have proposed that risk information can be more effectively conveyed using graphical and other types of visual display than by using more traditional numerical or verbal presentation formats, particularly for people with lower levels of literacy and numeracy (e.g. Gigerenzer and Edwards 2003). Visual displays have also been found to be beneficial for presenting information about low magnitude risks (e.g. Kaplan *et al.* 1985; Woloshin *et al.* 2000). According to Lipkus and Hollands (1999), visual displays have desirable properties that can enhance the understanding of risk information. For example, line graphs are particularly good for conveying trends in data (e.g. Meyer *et al.* 1997; Hollands and Spence 1998), whereas pie charts and bar charts are better for depicting proportions (Spence and Lewandowsky 1991; Hollands and Spence 1998). In addition, given a particular task, such as making a risk comparison, certain graphs allow the user to process information more effectively than when numbers are used in isolation (e.g. Kosslyn 1989). Lipkus and Hollands

(1999) also suggested that graphical displays are better at attracting and holding attention because they show information in concrete visual terms.

After reviewing evidence for the effectiveness of different types of display format, Lipkus and Hollands concluded that no single format will perform optimally in all situations. Rather, the effectiveness of a display will be affected by factors such as the display characteristics (e.g. use of colours, spacing), the conditions of presentation (e.g. lighting, time pressure), the complexity of the data, the particular task being carried out, the characteristics of the user and the particular performance measure selected. In line with this, Gigerenzer and Edwards (2003) recommended that doctors should use a range of pictorial representations to match the type of risk information that the patient most easily understands.

Line graphs, histograms, pie charts and icon displays

The most commonly used types of graphs are line graphs, bar charts and histograms, pie charts and icon displays. We will look at each of these in turn.

Line graphs

Line graphs have been shown to be particularly effective for communicating trends in data, such as survival or mortality rates and cumulative risks (see e.g. Mazur and Hickman 1993; Meyer *et al.* 1997). In such cases, for example, the magnitude of an event or events will be displayed (according to a scale shown on the vertical axis) over a series of points in time (as indicated on the horizontal axis). These are connected with a continuous line to show how the magnitude changes over time (see Figure 7.2). Line graphs allow readers to determine the rate of increase or decrease in the dependent variable (e.g. magnitude) as a function of changes in the independent variable (e.g. time), and are also useful for showing interactions between variables. In order to assess the utility of this form of presentation method, Mazur and Hickman (1993) examined how doctors, medical students and patients used line graphs to determine preference between alternative treatments. They found that the graphs provided enough information to assess patient preferences, although the patients differed from the doctors and students in terms of how they interpreted the curves.

Bar charts and histograms

Bar charts and histograms are often used to show relative risk rates (e.g. for people of different ages or sexes – see Figure 7.3). Thus, the level of risk (as indicated on the vertical axis) for the different comparison groups is shown in adjacent columns, and can be displayed separately as a function of some other factor, such as time period (on the horizontal axis). Several

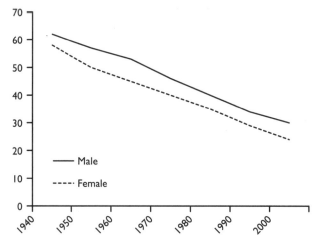

Figure 7.2   Example of a line graph showing the number of deaths from a fictitious disease

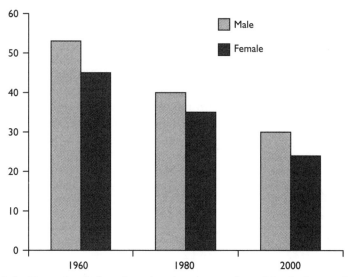

Figure 7.3   Example of a bar chart showing the number of deaths from a fictitious disease

studies have found that people find such displays helpful for understanding risk and that use of these displays can induce risk aversion compared with numerical forms of presentation. Stone *et al.* (1997), for example, found that people were prepared to pay more for safer products (toothpaste, tyres) when the associated risks were displayed on bar charts rather than numerically. More recently, Fortin *et al.* (2001) carried out a study to assess patient preferences for different ways of presenting information about risk of coronary heart disease, hip fracture and breast cancer, with and without HRT. They found that bar charts were preferred by 83 per cent of participants over line graphs, thermometer graphs, multiple face displays and survival curves. Focus group discussions revealed that bar charts were thought to be clearer and easier to understand. The study did not assess actual performance, however. It is interesting to note that some studies have shown that people prefer to have risk information displayed on bar charts than on other graphical formats or tables, even when use of the bar chart is not associated with more accurate interpretation of the displayed information (Edwards *et al.* 2002).

Pie charts

Pie charts are acknowledged to be particularly suited to conveying proportions rather than absolute amounts (e.g. Hollands and Spence 1998). Thus, such charts could be used to display the proportion of smokers and non-smokers who die from lung cancer each year or the proportion of males and females of different age groups who are injured in car accidents. A typical display consists of a circle with 'wedges' of different sizes being used to represent the comparison items. An example is shown in Figure 7.4. It should be noted, however, that not all studies have reported beneficial effects from using this form of display. Hampson *et al.* (1998), for instance, found that use of a pie chart failed to help convey the effects of smoking and radon exposure on lung cancer risk. In line with this, Fortin *et al.* (2001) noted that, in general, studies have shown pie charts to be less effective for

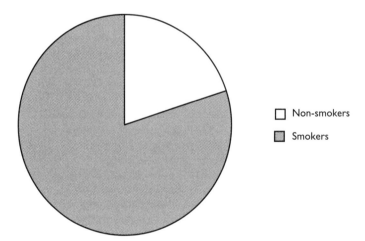

Figure 7.4   Example of a pie chart showing the proportion of smokers and non-smokers who died from lung cancer in 2000

conveying risk information (in terms of accuracy and speed of performance) than bar charts, histograms and numerical forms of presentation.

Icon displays

These come in various different forms, using various different types of icon, such as stick figures, faces, asterisks or dots. The basic idea is that information about frequencies or relative frequencies is indicated by the number of individual units displayed (see Figure 7.5). These displays have been used most extensively to aid relative risk judgements (Lipkus and Hollands 1999). Stone *et al.* (1997), for example, found that people were prepared to pay more for a safer product (i.e. were more risk averse) when the risk information was presented as stick figures rather than in numerical form. Subsequent experiments, using asterisks or faces rather than stick figures, have shown that the beneficial effect was due to the 'graphical nature' of the figures, rather than the 'humanizing' or 'discrete' nature of the stimuli. Although Stone *et al.* found beneficial effects of the stick figure display over the numerical format, there was no significant benefit of the stick figures over standard bar charts. In contrast, Elting *et al.* (1999) found that more correct decisions were made with icon displays than with tables, pie charts or bar charts. Their task involved doctors making decisions about whether to continue a (hypothetical) clinical trial or to suspend it so that additional (unplanned) statistical analyses could be carried out. Interestingly, despite the superior accuracy of the icon displays, none of the participants *preferred* this display format; in fact, the majority preferred the standard table format. Of the graphical displays tested, the majority preferred the bar chart.

Combined display formats

A number of studies have shown that combining visual displays with numerical and/or verbal information can affect several outcomes, such as

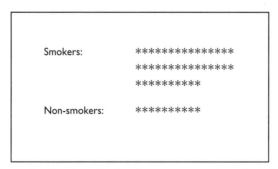

Figure 7.5 Example of an icon display showing proportion of smokers and non-smokers who died from lung cancer in 2000

perceived risk and the perceived helpfulness of the information. Hinks *et al.* (1998), for example, found that combined graphs and tables (which they called 'grables') produced fewer errors than use of graphs alone. They suggested that the grable form of quantitative display has the potential for communicating information across varied types of enquiry. However, the information must be displayed very clearly in order to be effective. The danger is that the display may appear cluttered as a result of too much information being presented, which may result in confusion and poorer performance.

The use of symbols, pictograms and pictographs

In addition to the types of visual display described above, individual visual symbols or pictograms/pictographs can be incorporated into printed information about risk and/or health. In general, symbols are not direct representations of the 'meaning' they are used to portray (e.g. a skull and crossbones to represent poison), whereas pictograms and pictographs are more direct representations, with the latter being used to represent more complex ideas (e.g. a person taking tablets with a glass of milk). As with other forms of visual display, one advantage of such symbols is that they should be more meaningful than written text to people with lower levels of literacy or non-native speakers of the dominant language in a country. In an experimental study, Houts *et al.* (1998) examined whether pictographs could enhance the recall of spoken medical instructions, such as 'rinse your mouth with baking soda after eating'. Students listened to lists of actions for managing fever and for managing a sore mouth, with one action list being accompanied by pictographs during both listening and recall. It was found that memory performance was significantly higher for the lists that were accompanied by pictographs (85 per cent as opposed to 14 per cent). However, given that the pictographs were re-shown at recall, it is not clear if they aided understanding of the information or had the potential to support longer-term memory. A follow-up study by Houts *et al.* (2001) found that a similar beneficial effect of pictographs was obtained when people with low levels of literacy were required to recall much larger amounts of medical information after a four-week delay. However, the pictographs were again re-shown at test, which limits the conclusions that can be drawn from the study.

One potential difficulty with the use of symbols or pictograms is selecting visual items that can be correctly and consistently interpreted by large numbers of people. Bernardini *et al.* (2000) therefore carried out an empirical study in which they asked people visiting pharmacies in a particular region in Italy to select which symbol best represented particular types of drug information (e.g. paediatric use, use in pregnancy, existence of side-effects, contraindications). They found that in the case of side-effects, paediatric use, use in pregnancy, and dose, most respondents produced consistent responses, whereas for therapeutic indications and contra-indications there was no uniformity in the answers. However, choices depended greatly on the level of education, age and employment status of the participants.

Use of computers to aid interpretation

Many types of display, including graphs and tables, can be easily produced by computers, particularly when the relevant information is already available in electronic form. Data can either be viewed on the computer or can be printed out, for example in the form of patient information leaflets. In the USA and Australia, most medicine information leaflets are generated online in community pharmacies at the time when patients collect or purchase their medicines. In terms of their utility for health professionals, Wright *et al.* (1998) suggested that computers have the advantage that they can help people, such as doctors, to make comparisons between different aspects of data, and can be used to display large amounts of complex data. They can also offer an expanded range of opportunities for flagging and automatic interpretation of numerical data (e.g. automated electro-cardiogram interpreters). However, Wright *et al.* pointed out that more advanced forms of computerized presentation often require users to undergo training before they can be used effectively. Currently, few doctors and other health professionals receive formal training and updates on the use of information technology, and this is not likely to change significantly in the short term.

Computers are being used increasingly in relation to patient education and communication, complementing traditional spoken and written leaflet-based approaches. Although few would argue that they are an effective replacement for personal contact from health professionals, there is evidence that they can play a useful complementary role. As Bental *et al.* (1999) noted, most patients find information access using a computer acceptable, given a suitably designed interface, and many find it less embarrassing accessing information in this way than by asking possibly trivial (and sometimes personal) questions of health professionals.

Using computers to tailor information

One potential advantage of using computers in relation to patient education is that they can facilitate the personalization or individualization of information (see e.g. Sellu 1987; Buchanan *et al.* 1995; McRoy *et al.* 1998; Cawsey *et al.* 2000). Sellu pointed out that a disadvantage of many written information leaflets is that they often contain some information that may not be relevant to a particular individual. One way of countering this is to produce different versions of a leaflet for different individuals, or groups of individual. However, this can be impractical in the case of written leaflets. Sellu therefore devised a computer program to generate personalised patient information. He assessed the usefulness of the generated leaflets by testing 115 hospital patients who had undergone a surgical operation, and found that 90 per cent reported the leaflets to be 'very useful'. In particular, the personalized nature of the leaflets was considered to be an important factor in making the patients read them and take note of their content.

At the simplest level, communications can be tailored by simply inserting a patient's name in a given slot to make a message appear more personal. However, at a more sophisticated level, they can be tailored by varying the context of the information, its order, or the way it is presented. The tailoring can be based on basic factual information such as age, sex, educational level, medical problem, or on a user's beliefs and attitudes. The majority of applications that have been developed to date have done the former. Cawsey et al. (2000), for example, developed and evaluated a personalized information system for patients with cancer. The system dynamically generated hypertext pages that explained diseases and treatments, using information in the patient's record as a basis for tailoring. A randomized control trial, comparing the system with a non-personalized one, showed significant results concerning patients' preferences for personalized information.

On a more general note, Kahn (1993) has pointed out that computer-generated leaflets can be stored, edited, updated, retrieved and printed on demand, and that the computer can readily accommodate the need for customization and personalization. Similarly, Kenny et al. (1998) suggested that computerized leaflets are an effective way of giving personalized information to patients in GP and other primary care settings, including pharmacies. Kenny et al. recommended that any author writing a new information leaflet intended for a wide audience should consider producing it in an electronic format in addition to any paper format.

As well as supporting patient education, computers have been used to calculate particular risks, and to aid doctors and other health professionals in risk management and treatment decisions. Hingorani and Vallance (1999), for instance, developed an interactive program for calculating cardiovascular risk in individual patients. They compared the program's performance with that of existing tables and guidelines, by means of hypothetical cases. They found that the program allowed more refined estimations of absolute and relative risk reductions from cholesterol-lowering drugs than the existing methods. They suggested that an additional advantage of the system is that it can be used during a consultation to allow the patient to see immediately the predicted health benefits of changes in lifestyle (e.g. stopping smoking) or drug treatments.

Computerized medical decision aids

A number of computerized decision aids have been developed over the past 20 years or so in order to support medical decision making. Decision aids differ from information aids in that they typically contain explicit components to help users clarify their values and incorporate these into the decision making process. According to Eysenbach (2000), computer-based applications have clear advantages over traditional media because of their interactive nature. Initially, the majority of decision aids were designed to help doctors and other health professionals to make decisions about patients' care (e.g. Medow *et al.* 2001). An advantage of such applications is that they can help doctors to integrate a patient's preferences (values) with scientific evidence, the patient history and local constraints (Eysenbach 2000). In recent years, however, we have also seen the development of medical decision aids aimed specifically at helping patients to make decisions about their treatments, and to support doctor–patient communications in relation to this. This section will focus on such patient decision aids and will assess the extent to which these could help, and have helped, patients weigh up the risks and benefits of different treatment options in order to select between them, or have helped them to understand the reasoning behind a doctor's recommendation or decision.

According to O'Connor and Edwards, patient decision aids prepare patients to participate with health care professionals in making deliberated, personalized choices about health care options, by enabling them to judge the relative value of the risks and benefits involved. They provide a framework in which treatment alternatives and their potential outcomes can be systematically analysed. Factors that should be considered in the treatment decision are outlined to a large extent in the context of individual patient characteristics. O'Connor and Edwards (2001: 220) noted that the general aim of patient decision aids is to help patients:

♦ understand the range of options available;
♦ understand the probable consequences of options;
♦ consider the value they place on consequences;
♦ participate actively with health professionals in deciding between options.

Following on from this, O'Connor *et al.* (2003) recommended that, as a general principle, decision support should respect a patient's values, personal resources and capacity for self-determination. The approach should include sharing power and responsibility based on a therapeutic alliance to reach an agreement about the problem, options, and the role in decision making. Thus, patients are helped to become involved in deliberating, planning and implementing the negotiated option.

Some aids are designed for patients to work through on their own, whereas others are developed for use during doctor–patient consultations.

The programs typically provide information in a highly interactive manner. Multiple formats of information, such as text, audio, still pictures and video are often provided. To date, patient decision aids have been developed for a range of situations, including medical therapies (e.g. for atrial fibrillation, low back pain and various cancers), diagnostic tests (e.g. amniocentesis), preventative therapies (e.g. hormone replacement therapy), clinical trial entry decisions and end-of-life decisions.

Man-Song Hing *et al.* (1999) developed a patient-centred decision aid to help patients with atrial fibrillation, who were considering anti-coagulant therapy, prepare for consultation. In using the aid, the patients reviewed key points about the risks of stroke and the benefits and risks of aspirin and warfarin. The information was tailored to take account of personal risk factors. Probability information was presented numerically and in an icon display. After reviewing the information, the patients completed a work-sheet that required their having to identify medical factors that would affect choice of outcome, attach values to the perceived risks and benefits of the different options, list any questions and then indicate their provisional preferences. The research team found that patients who used the aid were more prepared to make a treatment choice in the consultation than those in the control group.

A number of evaluation studies have been carried out in recent years to assess the utility of patient decision aids (e.g. O'Connor *et al.* 1999; Molenaar *et al.* 2000). In general, these evaluations have shown that use of such decision aids can have beneficial effects. For example, they have been shown to increase patient knowledge and reduce uncertainty, to create more realistic expectations, to reduce decisional conflict and to increase participation in decision making. However, there is less evidence that aids can alter and improve actual treatment choices, or improve patient satisfaction, and more systematic studies are needed in this area. One recent systematic evaluation, carried out by the Cochrane Review Team, assessed 34 randomized control trials conducted in the UK, USA and Canada and found that use of decision aids as adjuncts to counselling had superior effects on the quality of decisions compared with usual practices (O'Connor *et al.* 2003).

O'Connor and Edwards (2001) outlined a number of steps that need to be taken when developing and evaluating decision aids: assessing needs; assessing feasibility; identifying the decision support framework; selecting the methods of decision support; selecting the design and measures for evaluation; and planning dissemination. Thus, there is a need for a principled and systematic approach. Given recent trends, it seems likely that we will see a considerable increase in the availability of patient decision aids in the coming few years. It is important that these are systematically developed and properly evaluated if patient decision aids are going to play a useful role in patient-doctor communication and decision making.

The role of the internet in communicating information about risk and health

By far the most common use of computers in relation to risk and health at the present time is as a means of accessing the internet. Over the past 10 to 20 years the internet has become a global communication network that is accessed by millions of users. According to Hardey (1999), it is an interactive environment that transcends established national boundaries, regulations and distinctions between professions and expertise. Through use of the internet, increasing numbers of the general public and health care providers are able to gain free access to an expanding volume of information that was previously inaccessible. In this context, Levy and Strombeck (2002) noted that 'health and medicine' is the fourth most popular 'online subject' (after news, travel and weather), and that more than 20,000 different sites provide information on health and medical matters. Information about diseases (particularly allergies, cancer, heart disease, diabetes and digestive disorders), diet and nutrition, and drugs is most frequently sought. There is no evidence that the steady increase in usage is abating. Levy and Strombeck predicted that by the year 2005 the number of online health information seekers in the USA alone is expected to grow (from the current 52 million) to over 88 million. Within the UK, the Department of Health has anticipated a government internet resource 'Wired for Health' as a source of health information for schools, colleges and the public (Department of Health 1998).

As might be expected, there are both advantages and disadvantages to this vast increase in access to health-related information. On the positive side, the internet provides easy access to information on a large variety of health topics, which often includes recent research findings. It can lead to increased patient knowledge, which may result in early detection of particular ill-nesses. It can also benefit doctor–patient consultations by encouraging patients to participate more, and can lead to a reduction in unnecessary visits to the doctor for minor ailments. According to Jadad (1999), the internet will have a profound effect on the way patients and doctors interact, as it will 'foster a new level of knowledge among patients, enable them to have input into making decisions about their health care, and allow them to participate in active partnerships with various groups of decision makers' (p. 761). In addition, the internet can provide access to relevant disease-specific 'online communities' and self-care groups. In this context, Levy and Strombeck (2002) noted that one in four disease information seekers joins an online support group. Furthermore, for health professionals, the internet can be a valuable clinical tool, enabling them to exchange infor-mation with colleagues and patients, and to gain access to up-to-date clinical information.

Cassell *et al.* (1998) presented a theoretical rationale for using the internet to conduct persuasive public health interventions. They suggested that the internet provides a hybrid channel that combines the positive attributes of interpersonal communication and mass media channels. Specifically, internet-based resources have the capacity to provide the immediate trans-actional feedback that is necessary to induce behaviour change in a manner that is similar to that of interpersonal communication, but on a larger scale than has hitherto been possible. Thus, by soliciting information from users and by providing appropriate customized feedback, the internet can mimic the response-dependent quality of interpersonal communication. In this way, both source and message factors can be instantly and dynamically modified to realize the persuasive advantages associated with interpersonal channels. Following on from this, it should be possible to apply theories of health behaviour, such as the health belief model (see e.g. Rosenstock 1966) or the stages of change model (see e.g. DiClemente and Prochaska 1982) to internet communications in order to plan interventions that will bring about the desired effects on people's beliefs and health behaviours.

Unsurprisingly, however, there are also negative aspects associated with this vast growth in internet use. For instance, the increase in information access can lead to confusion and increased anxiety in users, particularly when conflicting information and advice is available. In addition, not all doctors are happy with patients becoming more proactive in their health care. Jadad (1999: 763) referred to the problem of clinicians 'finding them-selves upstaged by, and ill prepared to cope with, patients who bring along information downloaded from the Internet'. Similarly, Hardey (1999) pointed out that the internet represents a challenge to previous hierarchical models of information giving, with a shift in control – and a decline in awe (and sometimes trust) of doctors by patients.

Vetting and improving the quality of internet health sites

A major problem is that there is currently no formal 'vetting' of the infor-mation that is provided on internet sites, and it has been noted by pro-fessionals that a lot of the information is inaccurate and often misleading (see e.g. Jadad and Gagliardi 1998; Kim *et al.* 1999). As Jadad (1999: 762) noted, 'regardless of how powerful, fast or invisible technology becomes, the Internet will only be valuable in promoting efficient partnerships in health care if it delivers information that is relevant, valid, engaging and ready to apply'. Unfortunately, this is not currently the case. Berland *et al.* (2001), for example, reviewed a large number of US health information sites and found that many offer incomplete, misleading or difficult to understand information, or blur the distinction between providing advice and advertising their own products. McLeod (1998) pointed out that widespread access to such inaccurate, misleading and, in some cases, fraudulent informa-tion can pose a threat to public health. In this context, Eng (2001) suggested that the consequences of poor quality 'e-health' applications include 'inappropriate treatment or delays in seeking appropriate health care, damage to the patient-provider relationship, and violations of privacy and confidentiality (p. 12).

One reason for the wide variation in the quality of information available, as noted by Levy and Strombeck (2002), is that as things stand just about anyone can post information on the internet regardless of personal knowledge, qualifications or intentions. Thus, we need to heed Kenny and colleagues' warning that 'unless we evaluate the quality of clinical sites and their effects on users, we risk drowning in a sea of poor quality information' (1998: 473).

As a result of criticisms such as these, there have been several recent initiatives to guide the development and dissemination of 'high quality' health information on the internet. Several industrial and commercial organizations have produced codes of practice for ensuring information quality and reliability. Furthermore, several sets of guidelines and checklists have been developed to help users assess the information that is available. Kim *et al.* (1999), for instance, reviewed existing criteria that had been published for evaluating health-related information on the internet. They found that many authors did seem to agree on the key criteria, particularly in relation to content, design and aesthetics of a site and identified what they referred to as the top 12 quality criteria for evaluating health information on the internet. Following on from this study, Barnes *et al.* (2003) assessed the utility of these 12 key criteria. They found that 6 of the criteria, including content, design and aesthetics, currency of information and contact addresses, were significant predictors for selecting high-quality health information on the internet. However, compared to their perceived importance, participants' perceptions about information quality were not consistent when selecting quality websites. In addition, it should be noted that voluntary codes of practice and use of recommended evaluation criteria have obvious limitations. They may reduce, but will not prevent, users gaining access to unreliable information. Consensus still needs to be reached in relation to enforcement issues, as well as to more general ethical principles in relation to the internet. Furthermore, more needs to be done to develop effective strategies to increase the 'health literacy' of health information seekers, particularly for those with the greatest health care needs.

A critical issue in this respect is how to bridge the 'digital divide' and bring the internet and other health informatics to the people who have the highest need of them (Eysenbach 2000). As Eysenbach noted, although the 'information society' offers tremendous potential for reducing the knowledge gap between professionals and patients, it also brings a risk of widening the gap between those who have access to new technology and those who have been excluded. Clearly, this is an important issue that health professionals and policy makers will have to tackle in the coming years. If we fail to meet the current challenges that are being raised in relation to the internet, we may 'miss an extraordinary opportunity to make health care more efficient and equitable, moving instead into a health care environment ruled by confusion, battles of opinion, anxiety, and unnecessary conflicts' (Eysenbach 2000: 614). The final chapter of this book considers a number of other key issues that will need to be addressed if we are to deliver effective health information that can support improved doctor–patient communication and decision making, and improve health outcomes.

CHAPTER
8

Conclusions and future challenges

We started this book by looking at the 1995 'pill scare', and saw how what was thought to be a simple risk message issued by the CSM had unforeseen detrimental effects on a large number of women. One clear conclusion that was drawn from this was that combining uncertain information with dire consequences can (and probably will) frighten large numbers of people, especially if exacerbated by the media (Adams 1998). The 'pill scare' is not the only example of a 'poor risk communication' having a more detrimental effect on public health than the risks that it was trying to address. This final chapter will start by considering the question of why many risk communications fail to produce the expected (beneficial) effects. A number of the reasons have been touched on in the earlier chapters but will be brought together here. The chapter will then move on to look at what can, and should, be done to improve future risk communications. Much of this will involve setting out future challenges rather than offering ready-made solutions. Finally, the chapter discusses a number of ethical concerns that arise in relation to risk communication in health.

Why do so many risk communications fail?

There is no simple or 'single' answer to this question. Many communications do not have their intended effect because of a number of complex factors that typically interact with each other. These include the cognitive and emotional 'limitations' of the targeted recipients, the fact that people often vary in the values that they hold, the need to provide information for a mass audience that can nevertheless be made meaningful to individual recipients, and the problem that many people no longer trust a number of previously influential sources of risk messages.

Cognitive and emotional factors

A major reason why risk communications fail is because people simply do not understand the information they are given or because they misinterpret it in some way. We saw in Chapter 3 that many people are cognitively and/or emotionally ill-equipped to understand, retain and use risk information (Doyal 2001). We are all prone to a number of cognitive biases and are also influenced by the particular ways in which risk information is presented to us. These biases and influences affect the judgements of lay people and experts alike. Research has shown that the way in which information is presented affects how it is weighted in decisions. As Hibbard *et al.* (2002) pointed out, even very important attributes may not be used in decision making if information about them is not presented in such a way that it can be used effectively. Similarly, particular presentation formats, or forms of wording, can distort perceptions and judgements of risk. A major factor in the 'pill scare', for example, was the use of the phrase 'around twice the risk' when comparing second and third generation pills, without giving people any indication of the absolute (and very small) size of the actual risk levels. We also saw in Chapter 3 that many people have difficulty handling numerical information in general, particularly when presented as percentages (see e.g. Gigerenzer 2002). However, verbal frequency labels do not seem to provide an easy solution to the problem either. Numerous studies have shown that there is wide variability in the interpretation of terms such as '*rare*' or '*common*', even in a relatively restricted context (e.g. Mazur and Merz 1994; Timmermans 1994). Finally, we have also seen that, in addition to these cognitive factors, our judgements can be influenced by a number of emotional and affective factors, and that our 'feelings' can have a more influential effect than our cognitions on our judgements and behaviours (see e.g. Mellors 2000). Risk communicators need to be aware of, and attempt to take account of, all these limitations when deciding on the content and format of risk messages.

Values

Following on from these basic cognitive and emotional limitations, many of our emotional responses to risk information are also determined by the particular values that we hold. These different values will affect which particular aspects of risk will influence us most, and which sources of risk information will be trusted. Calman (1998) identified five basic human values with particular relevance to health and health care: autonomy, justice, beneficence, non-malevolence and utility. He pointed out that each is important but may be in conflict with the others. A key conflict in this respect is the tension that sometimes arises between the rights of an individual (i.e. autonomy) and the needs and rights of the population (i.e. justice and utility). This will be returned to at the end of this chapter. In addition to the five basic human values, Calman also noted that we need to take account of individual personal values, professional values, and societal and political values.

A significant factor when considering values is the relative importance that people attach to quality of life as opposed to longevity. It is often assumed that longevity is the appropriate outcome (and goal) for improved health. However, others might argue that quality of life may be just as important, or more so. In this context, Calman (1998) raised the question of the 'purpose of health' and whether it is simply a means to an end.

There is now a lot of evidence that people differ very much in the values that they hold and the meaning that they attach to particular risks. What might be thought of as a relatively unimportant risk to a health professional may be very significant as far as a patient is concerned, and vice versa. In one of our early studies (Berry et al. 1997), for example, we noticed that the younger people in our sample were extremely concerned about getting acne as a side-effect, whereas the doctors thought that this was relatively mild and inconsequential. Similarly, it has been noted that heroin addicts are not particularly concerned about the risks associated with frequent injections, often using dirty needles, as they value the 'positive' effects of the drug itself much more. It has been noted that, for some patients, particular side-effects are simply unacceptable and they refuse to expose themselves to even the smallest level of risk. Fraenkel et al. (2002), for example, reported that for many rheumatoid arthritis patients the risk of drug toxicity was unacceptable, even when reduced to a level that was far below the actual risk.

More generally, it has been observed that some people are absorbed by the risks inherent in the disease itself, whereas others are more concerned about the risks associated with any treatment, such as side-effects of medication, medical errors or becoming dependent on the doctor or hospital. In addition, specific risks will be weighed differently against each other and against what are seen to be the potential benefits of the treatment. Furthermore, the values that we hold will also influence how we think about the perceived benefits of any treatment, thus affecting how they are weighed against the risks in any particular case. Clearly, this means that we need to know about the particular value systems that people hold in order to develop communications that take account of these.

Mismatch between population-based information and individual needs

Another reason why risk communications can fail is because there is a mismatch between risk information that is based on population statistics and the needs of particular individuals to apply this information to their own circumstances. Thus, as we saw in Chapter 3, experts tend to base their judgements and communications on population-derived evidence. However, most lay people are only concerned about their individual level of risk, and the particular way in which they will be affected. Remember the quote from the patient who asked what it means to have a 5 per cent risk of stroke? In his eyes, the risk was either 0 or 100 per cent; he would either have a stroke or not (see Chapter 3). In addition, many people see themselves as being different from the average person, which can lead them to downplay or ignore generic risk messages. These differences in perspective will also influence people's uptake of recommended treatments and preventative measures, such as being vaccinated. A challenge for risk communicators is therefore to make risk information derived from population statistics meaningful to individual recipients of the message. People's understandable 'egocentrism' can lead to what is known as the 'prevention paradox' (see e.g. Rose 1985). This is where a prevention measure (such as vaccination), that brings much benefit to the population as a whole, may be seen to offer little obvious benefit to each participating individual. Furthermore, any perceived individual benefit may well be outweighed by any associated perceived risks, reducing the likelihood that people will engage in the recommended behaviour. We have witnessed a clear example of this in recent years, in that many patients have not wanted their babies to be given the combined Measels, Mumps and Rubella (MMR) vaccine.

Trust

Even if risk messages are understood and interpreted appropriately, and can be made meaningful to individuals, the recipients will not necessarily take account of them and follow the recommended advice if they do not trust the information in the message or the source of the information. Unfortunately, in many risk communication situations, the communicator and recipient neither understand nor trust each other (Fox and Irwin 1998). Fox and Irwin reasoned that if a speaker and listener differ greatly in terms of prior beliefs, social status, experience with the risk and world view, then communication is unlikely to resemble the smooth transfer of probability information. Furthermore, if a risk has been discussed at length among various listeners, as is often the case with politically-charged risks, then it is likely that polarization will have taken place and that listeners will be less amenable to updating their beliefs.

As Bennett (1998) pointed out, in most instances risk messages are judged first and foremost by the source, rather than the content; that is, who is telling me this and can I trust them? If the answer is 'no', the message is likely to be disregarded no matter how accurate, well-intentioned and well-delivered. Unfortunately, many sources of risk information are distrusted. Experts no longer command automatic trust, no matter how genuine their expertise (see e.g. Bennett 1998). Some people prefer to rely on the advice of family and friends, feeling that such people will be honest with them (even in cases where these significant others do not have the necessary 'knowledge' to provide an informed opinion). According to

Calman (2001: 1328), trust is the force that binds patient and doctor: 'Lose the trust of your patient and suspicions and concerns arise. Ensure that the patient knows that what you do, what you advise and the language you use are in his or her best interests, and the trust developed will be a powerful and therapeutic force'. He warned that once trust is lost, it is difficult to regain; the key aim of the doctor must be to develop and maintain trust.

What can be done to improve risk communications?

One might feel from reading the preceding sections that we are facing a hopeless task and that, in many instances, it might be better to revert to providing people with little or no relevant risk information. In the case of medicine and other health treatments, this would mean returning to the old paternalistic model of doctor–patient communication. However, this solution seems to be rather drastic. As we have seen in Chapters 5 and 6, there is plenty of evidence that people do want to receive risk information, and that it is important that they understand the information they are given in order to play an effective part in shared decision making and to provide fully informed consent. According to Bennett and Calman (1999), the main purpose of risk communication is not to defuse public concern or avoid action, but to produce an informed public that is involved, reasonable, thoughtful and collaborative. Risk communications will be effective if they alert the target audience (either an individual or the wider population) as to what is the hazard, the extent of the danger, and what should be done about it. Thus, simply not providing the information is not a realistic or acceptable solution to the problem.

General strategies

In recent years, various risk communication 'strategies' have been advocated by researchers and risk consultants. In terms of communicating numerical information, Paling (2003) made the following set of recommendations:

♦ avoid using descriptive terms only;
♦ use standardized vocabulary that is agreed by colleagues at local and national level;
♦ use a consistent denominator (i.e. 1 in 1000 and 10 in 1000, not 1 in 1000 and 1 in 100);
♦ offer positive and negative outcomes;
♦ use absolute numbers;
♦ use visual aids for probabilities.

Furthermore, Paling stressed that three important developments are needed in order for effective risk communication to improve the quality of health care. First, doctors need more training in communicating risks to patients.

Second, more research is needed on how different strategies, particularly the use of visual aids, help patients to understand risk. Finally, research should assess how differences in culture, age and gender affect patients' perceptions of risks. In relation to training, Paling noted that in other industries where risks have to be conveyed to the public (e.g. chemical, nuclear and food industries) usually only a few specially-trained people carry out the task on behalf of their organizations. In contrast, in health care, almost every doctor who interacts with patients has to communicate risk information, yet few have had any training.

In terms of more general risk strategies, Calman (2001: 1327) endorsed Gutteling and Wiegman's (1996) list of recommendations, which is as follows:

♦ The communication's goal and intentions should be clearly described in the message.
♦ Risk information must not be misleading – i.e. it must be verifiable and presented in agreement with the scientific state of the art.
♦ If there are scientific doubts, the public should be made aware of them.
♦ Risk information should be complete – it is important not to delete any relevant information.
♦ Risk comparisons, especially numerical or statistical information, must be used cautiously.

However, rather than providing an instant panacea, this list can be viewed as raising as many questions as it answers. Thus, most people would agree that the public needs to be made aware of scientific doubts, but how can this be done most effectively? We know that people have particular difficulty dealing with uncertainty. Similarly, in relation to the suggestion that risk information should be complete, in many instances there is simply too much 'relevant' risk information that could be provided to people. The question then becomes, how do you decide which information should be included and what should be omitted? Furthermore, few researchers and practitioners working in this area would disagree with the suggestion that risk information should not be misleading, but we know that there are subtle, and sometimes unintentional, ways that people might be misled (e.g. by framing the information in particular ways, or by providing certain types of comparative information), in addition to outright falsehoods. It is also the case that the above list of recommendations omits some key points. For example, the list does not include the statement that, wherever possible, risk information should be evidence-based. Similarly, it is vital that risk messages and their effects are evaluated in order to ensure that the recipients of any message will understand the information and act on it in the manner intended by the communicator. Again, there is no mention of this. In making these points, it is not that I am arguing against Gutteling and Wiegman's recommendations. Indeed, despite their limitations, they are useful general principles which could and should be applied. One simply needs to recognize that they are only a sensible starting point, and that adherence to them will not necessarily guarantee effective risk communication.

In Chapters 6 and 7 we saw that other researchers have advocated the use of more specific one-off solutions, such as tailoring messages to individuals, using a 'standardized language of risk' or presenting information in multiple formats, as a means of improving risk communications. As we will see in the sections that follow, however, although these suggestions offer some promise, they are not all problem-free, particularly in relation to their likely impact in the short term.

Tailoring messages to individuals

Gutteling and Wiegman (1996) proposed that a principal 'ground rule' of risk communication is that the information should be customized to the receiver's needs. They identified three aspects of this. First, the information that is provided should address questions that are relevant to the receiver, as opposed to addressing irrelevant or never-asked questions. Second, the information must be comprehensible and not add to further confusion. Finally, the new information should be presented adequately, for example with a logical structure, and reinforced with textual aids. Other researchers have further developed the notion of customizing or tailoring information to particular users or sub-groups of users.

In terms of medicine information leaflets, the majority of materials that are available are currently not tailored to particular sub-groups of the population or to individuals. In recent years, however, a number of researchers have argued in favour of such tailoring (e.g. Skinner *et al.* 1999; Kreuter and Holt 2001; Straus 2002). After reviewing the literature to date, Skinner *et al.* (1999) suggested that tailored print communications are generally better read and remembered than generic communications, and that there is also evidence that they are more effective for influencing behaviour change. Campbell *et al.* (1994), for instance, compared the effects of tailored versus non-tailored printed physician recommendations for dietary change in nearly 500 family practice participants. They found that the tailored communications resulted in significantly higher message recall and also led to a significantly greater reduction in dietary fat intake (23 per cent compared to 9 per cent in the 'non-tailored' group). Similarly, Marcus *et al.* (1996) found that tailored exercise promotion materials resulted in significantly increased exercise levels (being active for at least 30 minutes, five days per week) in healthy sedentary men and women, compared with non-tailored materials.

Tailored systems have now been developed in several medical domains, including asthma, diabetes, migraine, cancer and dental treatments. The particular goal of the systems also varies to include supporting patient decision making, providing information to aid management of chronic conditions, diagnostic advice and health promotion (Bental *et al.* 1999).

Individually-tailored communication efforts use data gathered about individual characteristics to design and present personalized health promotion messages to individuals that match each person's unique background and orientation (Rimer and Glassman 1997). As Kreuter *et al.* (1999) noted, however, full tailoring of even a relatively short communication to individuals could result in hundreds of thousands of possible different messages being needed, which may well not be cost-effective. Although computer generation of materials will help to some extent (see e.g. Sellu 1987 and Chapter 7), a key issue that remains to be addressed is: how much tailoring is needed to produce a significant benefit? Berry (in press) recently suggested that a potential compromise between the two extremes (generic as opposed to individually-tailored messages) might be to produce leaflets for particular sub-groups of the population (e.g. elderly patients or parents of young children), if these can be shown to be beneficial. In this respect, Kreuter *et al.* (1999) also distinguished between targeted generic materials that are intended for a particular sub-group of the population and designed to take account of the specific needs and concerns of that sub-group, and fully tailored materials that are intended to reach a specific individual and have been derived from an individual assessment. They suggested that both types of material could contribute to individual behaviour change in a positive way. Future research needs to identify the circumstances in which targeted generic materials are likely to be beneficial and those in which it would be necessary to produce fully tailored messages in order to have the desired impact. As Kreuter *et al.* noted, 'there are clearly many ways of tailoring materials, many ways to deliver such materials, and many possible responses to such materials' (1999: 281).

Kreuter *et al.* have also pointed out that there is a strong public health rationale for tailoring materials, and that computer-tailored health communications should be viewed as a tool of public health communicators, to be incorporated into comprehensive programmes of health promotion, disease prevention and disease management. They suggested that the traditional public health approach of using mass media to disseminate health information could eventually be supplanted with what they term 'mass customization' – that is, allowing the fine-tuning of message content to suit particular needs but on the scale of mass communication. It is likely that in future years we will see a growing use of such communication methods.

A standardized language of risk?

As Breakwell (1997) noted, several researchers have been tempted to look for some means of standardizing risk information in order to facilitate communication. A frequently suggested means of doing this has been to use some simple linear index of risk, akin to the Richter scale, that allows novel and unfamiliar hazards to be rated relative to risks that people have already learned to evaluate. As was seen in the previous chapter, one problem with this is that it is difficult to select comparison items whose probability of occurrence is known and agreed upon by large numbers of people. For instance, how many people live in the average country, or are murdered in the UK each year? In Chapter 6 we saw two examples of simple standardized scales that do not include comparison items: the EC recommended terms for describing the probability of medication side-effects, and Calman's (1996) Verbal Risk scale. Unfortunately, neither scale was developed on the basis of empirical evidence, and both have been shown to lead to a considerable overestimation of the risk of side-effects by lay people, patients and doctors. Use of these scales has also been shown to result in judgements of increased risk to health and reduced intention to take the medication, compared with equivalent numerical presentations of risk (see Berry *et al.* 2003c for a review of the relevant studies).

As a result of these findings, and others, we have questioned the feasibility and value of using such standardized scales, at least in the short term. Like Edwards and Elwyn (2001b), we have pointed out that standardizing the language does not allow the flexibility required for dealing with people with different levels of literacy, numeracy, and attitudes (Berry *et al.* 2003). Edwards and Elwyn argued that 'the nature of risk, its burden, the context and the timeframe over which one has to live with it, are all important determinants of how individuals interpret risk for themselves, and of whether they choose to accept it' (2001: 260). In addition, we know that we cannot easily separate consideration of the size of risk from the value attached to harm; that is, its meaning and implications for a person's life. Similarly, as we have seen, we should not think about the risks associated with particular treatments in isolation from the likely beneficial effects. In medicine taking, for example, there is normally only a single benefit that is sought, but the potential risks are often multiple (Edwards *et al.* 1996).

The problem of context

There is now considerable evidence to show that risk judgements are influenced by the particular context in which they occur. As Fox and Irwin (1998) argued, the social, informational, motivational and discourse context in which beliefs are constructed and statements are formulated provides a myriad of additional cues that influence what is expressed by speakers and what is understood by listeners. Context can be provided, for instance, by the characteristics of the stimulus domain, the perceiver's knowledge and experience, the goal of the communication, the way information is framed, the presence of multiple alternatives or the way probabilities are presented (Verplanken 1997). In terms of effects on probability judgements, Weber and Hilton (1990) found that probability judgements were influenced by the severity of the event outcome, with lower estimates being given in relation to 'likely' number of murders, for example, than to 'likely' number of injuries (see Chapter 3). More recently, my own research group carried out two experiments to investigate how people's perception of risk and intended health behaviours were affected by whether a medicine was prescribed for themselves or for a young child (Berry in press). In both experiments we found that both parents and non-parents perceived risk to be higher, and said that they would be less likely to take (or give) the medicine when the recipient was a child. They also produced significantly higher probability estimates when interpreting the EC recommended term '*common*' when the medicine was prescribed for a child.

Standardized scales for professionals

Our scepticism about the use of standardized risk scales with the general public is also shared by many health professionals. Edwards *et al.* (1998), for example, asked a number of different primary care professionals for their views of such scales, and found that the majority expressed considerable reservations. In particular, the health professionals were very pessimistic about the likelihood that patients would find use of standardized terms helpful, as they felt that such generic solutions would not capture many aspects of the communication process (such as non-verbal elements, mental images, past experience and discussion about the meaning of risk to individual patients). Despite this scepticism, the primary care professionals were much more optimistic about the use of such scales in communication between professionals, both within and between disciplines (see also Edwards *et al.* 2001). The participants felt that this would enable them to be more consistent in their appreciation of the risks of certain illnesses, complications, procedures and treatments, and to be more uniform in *what* they were trying to convey to patients, rather than *how*. In line with this, Tavana *et al.* (1997) reported on the successful implementation of a standardized set of risk phrases within an expert (financial analyst) community.

Some support for the suggestion that standardized scales might be more appropriate for use with professional groups comes from our studies, where we tested doctors' interpretations of the EC and Calman verbal descriptors (Berry *et al.*, submitted). Although the doctors significantly overestimated the likelihood of side-effects occurring when given the verbal descriptors (as did our general population and student samples), the amount of variability in their responses was much lower than that shown by the non-medically qualified participants, raising the potential for use of a shared language. Of course, if this restricted use of standardized terms is shown to be beneficial, then it is possible that extending their use to the wider population might be achieved in the longer term. However, this would require an effective and extensive education programme, where people would be trained, for instance, that when a side-effect is said to be 'common' this means that it will occur in only 1 to 10 per cent of the people taking the medicine.

Additional problems

Another problem with simple linear risk scales is that many hazards can be characterized on several dimensions, such as controllability and predictability as well as magnitude. As Breakwell (1997) noted, this makes it very difficult to compare risks on any uni-dimensional scale. Instead, Breakwell advocated using an N-dimensional scaling approach. However, this would require consensus about which dimensions should be used, and about the location of each hazard on each dimension. It would then be necessary to establish an intelligent iconography to represent the different dimensions. Finally, as with the extension of any standardized uni-dimensional scale to the general public, widespread use of multi-dimensional scales would require considerable investment in a public education programme. Such mass education programmes would have to be aimed at risk communicators, regulators, policy makers and the media, in addition to lay people, if we want to ensure that future risk messages conform to the 'selected standardized means of communication'. In line with this, Sless (2001: 558) argued that if we are to improve the quality of health information for the patient, we must address the training needs of those who regulate health information, and those who produce the information: 'We need a new generation of regulators, familiar with information design principles, who can create regulations that encourage good design rather than inhibit it'.

Presenting risk information in multiple formats

Another suggested way of improving risk communication has been to present the information in more than one form or format. For example, a number of authors (e.g. Edwards *et al.* 2001; Schechtman 2002) have pointed out the limitations and biasing effects of describing risk reductions simply in 'relative' terms (such as there being 'twice the level of risk' of thrombosis for users of third generation oral contraceptives), particularly where the absolute probability levels are very low (as they were in the 'pill scare'). These researchers have therefore advocated that risk reductions should be communicated using both relative and absolute forms of presentation. Edwards *et al.* (2001: 3), for example, proposed that 'researchers should present results with both relative and absolute risk estimates and not present either in isolation, which may be misleading or insufficiently helpful for arriving at a decision'. They argued that such methods are 'nearer to the whole truth'.

Similarly, several researchers (e.g. Weber and Hilton 1990) have suggested that given the limitations associated with both verbal and numerical forms of presenting risk information, we should use appropriate combinations of the two types of information, building on the advantages of each method. Others working in the area have advocated supplementing this, where possible, with graphical representations in order to make the information more meaningful for people with lower levels of literacy, or who do not speak the native language of a country (e.g. Kaplan *et al.* 1985; Woloshin *et al.* 2000; Gigerenzer and Edwards 2003).

Finally, other researchers and practitioners have argued that we should not give people information about the risks of potential treatments without also telling them about the likely benefits (including the risks of not undertaking treatment). Both Amery (1999) and Vander Stichele *et al.* (2002) have pointed out that a limitation of the current EC guidelines, and the ensuing legislation, is the emphasis on risk and the absence of information about the benefits of the medicine. Amery (1999) argued that adequately informing patients about the benefits as well as the risks of treatments would not only improve patients' knowledge about their medicines and improve compliance, but would also improve safety management. In addition, he suggested that patients will be more able to deal with adverse effects if they are adequately informed about the likelihood, characteristics and expected time course of these events, as well as about measures that will help prevent or relieve them. Vander Stichele *et al.* (2002) recommended that benefit messages for branded packages should be standardized and tested at the generic level. They suggested that adding benefit information to leaflets will enable patients to reach a more balanced judgement, and heighten the value of the patient package insert as an instrument of regulatory policy.

In each of the above cases, however, the recommended 'improvement' involves increasing the absolute amount of information that would need to be communicated. This could easily result in an 'information overload' and cause confusion. In the case of medication side-effects, for example, many medicines are associated with a large number of side-effects. If we present information about all of these (in addition to information about the likely benefits of taking the medicine *and* the risks of not taking it, using relative and absolute formats), in numerical, verbal and graphical form, then the resulting explanation is likely to be very lengthy and potentially confusing. Indeed, one wonders how small the print on the patient package insert would need to become in order to cover the information on a single sheet of paper.

Preliminary recommendations

It should be clear from the above discussion that we will need to be selective about which information to present in risk communications, and in which formats, for particular audiences. Some general recommendations in this context were noted in Chapter 6. For example, in relation to medicines, it is fairly widely acknowledged that the minimum information that patients need to be given should cover the medicine's name and purpose, details of dosage and how it should be taken, and any special precautions and adverse effects. The content needs to be correct, balanced and unbiased. However, it is clear that further research is needed about the effects of different formats on different audiences, before detailed recommendations can be produced. In the meantime, we should remember that, whatever specific forms or formats are adopted as 'best practice' and incorporated into future guidelines, we need to ensure that the development of new materials takes account of patient information needs, is based on up-to-date scientific evidence, and that it is designed in line with professional advice (Sless 2001). In addition, the materials should be user tested and refined until they meet agreed benchmark performance standards. As Sless (2001) noted, if this is not done, health professionals would be prudent neither to use the information, nor endorse it, and to advise patients that they will be at risk if they use it. This view is in line with Gutteling and Wiegman's (1996) proposals that risk communications must be based on a systematic planning process. Indeed, they conceptualized risk communication as 'the systematic planning of information transfer based on scientific research, to prevent, solve or mitigate the risk problem with adjusted and customised information (risk messages) for specific target groups' (p. 42). Gutteling and Wiegman identified a number of steps in their systematic planning approach, including policy preparation, development of a risk communication strategy, conducting necessary research into the risk event and public opinions, designing a communication plan, implementing the results and evaluating the outcomes against established goals. Calman (2001) also included 'careful planning' in his list of essential factors in relation to effective risk communication. Other factors included the importance of credible sources of advice, openness, sharing uncertainty, the need to accept the public as partners, listening to concerns, coordinating with other credible sources and the importance of meeting the needs of the media.

It can be seen from Gutteling and Wiegman's and Calman's lists that there is more to effective risk communication than just getting the content of the message and its manner of presentation right. There also need to be appropriate policies, regulations and training programmes in place to ensure that the messages are generated in accordance with the established 'best practice' and that people are appropriately prepared to convey and receive the information. As we noted earlier, effective training programmes will not simply be needed to educate the general public but will also need to extend to relevant health professionals, policy makers, regulators, designers and the media. In a similar vein, Bennett et al. (1999: 207) stressed that although formulating a risk message and presenting it effectively remain essential, these are only part of the overall effort: 'Risk management that overlooks stakeholders' basic concerns cannot usually be saved by good communication techniques late in the day'.

Ethical concerns

So far this chapter has looked at why so many risk communications fail to produce the desired effects, and has considered a number of ways in which communications can be improved. Much of the discussion here, and in the earlier chapters, has been concerned with the questions of what information should be presented to consumers, and in which particular form or format, as well as some of the broader implications for developing necessary training programmes, regulations and policies. Effectively addressing questions and issues such as these presupposes that we are clear about the overall purpose or goal of the communication. Yet, this often involves taking account of a number of ethical considerations. For example, some people might believe that the overall goal of risk communication should be to inform decision making, whereas others might equally strongly believe that the primary goal should be to influence behaviour. Related to this is the fact that, in many situations, we do not necessarily know, or agree, what a satisfactory outcome of a particular risk communication would be. As Calman (2001: 47) questionned, is it 'full public information, the avoidance of exposure to a risk, no public outcry, or more research being generated'? This section considers a number of more general questions and ethical concerns that arise in relation to risk communication in health. At the outset we should note that these ethical considerations typically raise a number of questions to which no easy answers are available.

As Jungermann (1997) pointed out, informing people about risks related to health or other aspects of life can, and does, pose ethical dilemmas for the communicator. Whatever form of content of information is chosen, one or other ethical principle (such as honesty, altruism, autonomy, equity or fairness) is likely to be violated. Both ethically and legally, the principle of autonomy of the individual is central to medical ethics (Markham 1998). Autonomy is the right for adults to decide for themselves what they want to do. However, as yet, there is no general agreement in our society about when the objective of risk communication should be to inform people so that they can make their own (autonomous) choices, and when it should be to 'manipulate' them so as to induce a desired behaviour. Morgan and Lave (1990), for example, suggested that although it is probably all right to 'manipulate' behavior when people are faced by an immediate life-threatening danger (such as an impending tornado), there is much less agreement about the legitimacy of trying to change behaviour in the face of less immediate risks (such as smoking or practising unprotected sex).

Edwards (2003) recently noted that, with shifts towards greater autonomy for patients, the goal of risk communication is changing from one of simply trying to improve the population's health to one of informing people, enabling them to make their own choices, regardless of whether this reduces risk. This may lead to 'informed dissent', which may in turn produce tensions between what is perceived to be good for populations and what individuals perceive to be good for themselves. We may need to accept that increased involvement by patients (and risk communication as a means towards this) may therefore be based more on values than on evidence.

The question of autonomy

Schneider (1998) distinguished between two 'ideal' types of autonomy: the optional model and the mandatory model. According to the former position, the moral doctrine of informed consent entitles, but does not require, a patient to take an active role in decision making regarding treatment. Schneider further posited that the optional autonomist believes that patients should be helped to address individual or structural barriers that prevent them from making decisions about treatments but, at the end of the day, accepts that people may not want to exercise their autonomy in medical matters to the full. Indeed, he recognized that people may have good reasons for not wanting to participate fully in decision making and that, in general, the elderly and those who are most seriously ill are the least likely to want to make their own medical decisions. Thus, people might feel less competent than doctors or just too debilitated, or they might simply want to be 'manipulated' into a course of action that they actually want to pursue but, for some reason, have been resisting.

In contrast, the mandatory model holds that people need to exercise their autonomy and must do so. Thus, according to Schneider, 'the mandatory autonomist favours a view of autonomy that makes it practically unwise and morally objectionable for the patient to forswear making medical choices personally' (1998: 10). Schneider presented four arguments that can be used to justify this position: the prophylaxis argument (that doctors cannot be trusted to overcome their own self interests); the therapeutic argument (that patients who control their own treatments will be restored more quickly to health); the false consciousness argument (that patients really want to exert control but have been prevented from doing so by doctors); and the moral argument (that people have a moral duty to make the choices that shape their lives).

Finally, Schneider noted a further complicating factor, in that medicine is becoming increasingly institutionalized so that medical decisions are increasingly made in a bureaucracy and in times of economic stringency. He argued that the central dilemma is that while patients, diseases, treatments, doctors and hospitals all vary greatly, legal rights, legislative and judicial principles, administrative regulations, institutional rules and social policies all depend on generalization.

Ethical dilemmas for individuals

Morgan and Lave (1990) distinguished ethical dilemmas that exist on an individual level from those that occur at an institutional and societal level.

To illustrate ethical dilemmas that can occur at an individual level, they considered the question of how a genetic counsellor or doctor should inform a patient about the risks of having a handicapped child when a positive test result is received. The question is difficult to answer as the information that needs to be conveyed is complex and because the health professionals will undoubtedly have their own values with respect to raising handicapped children as opposed to undergoing a therapeutic abortion. Thus, to what extent should doctors and counsellors be open with patients and let them know their personal views, and to what extent should they be trying to respect the patient's autonomy? Should they frame the information that they present to patients in a negative or positive way, knowing that whichever wording they choose is likely to influence the patient's reactions to some extent? In many circumstances, health professionals are advised to try to be fair by presenting 'both sides of a coin', but offering multiple perspectives is not without its problems and may well add to patient confusion.

Similar ethical issues arise in relation to screening. For example, as Markham (1998) has questioned, whose interests are central in pre-implantation screening – the embryos' or those of the future parents? Should we screen in-utero for incurable diseases that will not be realized for 40 years? Currently, the criteria for a screening programme are that it must be in the interests of all individuals screened, it should be targeted at a particular problem, it should yield an accurate result, an effective treatment should be available, and that it should be cost-effective (Markham 1998). Clearly, however, interpreting and using such criteria is not straightforward. Furthermore, it is becoming apparent that, with medical and scientific advances such as the Human Genome Project, these difficulties will increase. Indeed, it is likely that we will soon be provided with choices that would have been inconceivable to any previous generation.

Patients' attitudes to risk vary in that some are prepared to accept a small risk of an early death in return for a high probability of a longer life. Others, however, may prefer not to face even a small risk of an early death but would rather accept it when it comes, even if it might be earlier than if a particular treatment were undertaken. Similarly, attitudes differ in relation to the value placed on length of life as opposed to quality of life, with some people refusing to have treatments that disrupt their lives in the short term, in the hope of a longer-term cure.

Ethics and informed consent

An area that has raised particular ethical concerns is seeking and providing informed consent. As we saw in Chapter 5, eliciting proper informed consent is one of the most demanding challenges that doctors face. The General Medical Council in the UK stipulates that patients must be given sufficient information, in a form that they can understand, in order to enable them to make informed decisions about their care. However, studies have shown that many doctors treat informed consent as little more than a ritual (e.g. Edwards *et al.* 1998). Hall (2001) distinguished between fulfilling the 'legal obligation' in relation to disclosing the necessary information and meeting the 'moral obligation' to make sure that patients understand the information. In this respect, doctors need to ensure that patients have not only heard and understood what they have been told, but that they are competent to reason about the alternative courses of action and that they are acting voluntarily. However, questions still remain in relation to how much information needs to be conveyed and how doctors can best ensure that patients have understood what they have been told and that they are competent to make an informed decision. Doyal (2001) has recently argued that, even though many studies have shown that patients often have cognitive and emotional difficulties when understanding clinical information, this should not undermine their potential to provide full informed consent. Rather, she suggested that more attention will have to be paid to improving patient information materials and doctors' communication skills. In addition, Doyal pointed out that cognitive and emotional inequality among patients is often a reflection of wider social and economic inequalities, and that these will also need to be addressed.

Institutional and societal issues

In addition to ethical issues that arise at the individual level, Morgan and Lave (1990) noted the types of ethical problem that can occur at the institutional and societal level, and the need to consider organizational and social factors in relation to these. As an example, they raised the question of whether companies should be made to label all goods fully (e.g. referring to the use of genetically engineered products) even when they know that this might deter some people from purchasing or consuming them and from deriving a known benefit. Should organizations be compelled to inform people about very small risks, even when some people do not want to be informed and some may even be harmed as a result? In the case of screening, should a less effective procedure for a relatively common condition take priority (when resources are limited) over a very effective procedure for a much rarer condition? To date, policy makers have tended to make such choices by adopting the principle of 'the greatest good for the greatest number of people'.

A necessary part of the process is to take account of the benefits of any health treatment or programme and, in some way, balance them against the risks which will be reduced. In this context, a distinction can be made between cost-benefit analysis and cost-effectiveness analysis (British Medical Association 1990). In the former case, the decision is typically whether to spend money to save lives; that is, to attempt to weigh lives against sums of money, a process that raises enormous ethical concerns.

In contrast, cost-effectiveness analysis makes the assumption that resources are available, even if limited, and is used to help make decisions about how best to limit the risk concerned. As the British Medical Association (1990) noted, given that risks to health are of two kinds (to length of life and to quality of life), there is interest in making rationing fairer by combining these elements to produce an overall measure of benefit. The Association argued that this helps in making choices, for example, between spending a given sum on a few expensive operations designed to increase length of life and a lot of less expensive operations designed to increase quality of life.

Regulators and policy makers also have to make decisions about when to ban particular substances and hazards in order to eliminate the associated risks. As noted in Chapter 2, however, it is not feasible or sensible to argue that all risks should be eliminated. Most activities, technologies and substances are associated with some risks, and to ban them could actually result in a greater level of harm than the original risk would have produced. Inman (1986), for example, calculated that if all drug risks were eliminated our average life expectancy would only be increased by some 37 minutes. But if this was achieved by banning all effective medicines and vaccines, then the costs would be an average loss of life expectancy of 10 to 20 years.

Clearly, there is some risk in almost everything we do. Thus, the British Medical Association (1990) proposed that risks which we face involuntarily as a result of public decision making and administration are best managed in a climate of the highest public awareness possible. Risks which we face at a personal level are most effectively managed by us as individuals provided that we know what the risks are and how they compare with each other. In a similar vein, Calman (2002) proposed three principles in relation to risk communication and public policy that should guide decision making and communication. He recommended that the public has a right to know the evidence on which decisions are based, that if they disagree with the policy then they should be aware of the consequences of their decision, and finally that individuals should not be allowed to opt out of some aspects of health and safety. Clearly, many of the issues that arise at the institutional and societal level are likely to be complex and will require multi-level solutions, involving a range of stakeholders. Inevitably, many of these issues will remain a challenge to us over the coming decade.

Concluding comments

We have seen throughout this book that effective risk communication is crucial if we want to improve health. We have also seen, however, that achieving this is far from easy or straightforward. Many people are not well equipped, either cognitively or emotionally, to understand complex probabilistic information and to apply it to their own circumstances. Despite the fact that several researchers and practitioners have advocated various 'advances' in communication methods, including specially devised scales and techniques, we are still far from clear how best to communicate risk information in health. Indeed, many of the recommended 'advances' have not been shown to lead to the promised benefits, and some have raised other broader problems, for example in relation to ethical questions.

However, we should not be too pessimistic. We know far more about how *not* to communicate information concerning risk than we did ten years ago, and we are making definite progress towards establishing how we can best communicate risk in order to bring about the desired positive effects, while avoiding or reducing unnecessary and unanticipated negative effects. Furthermore, given advances in our scientific methods and knowledge, we are likely to see considerably more progress over the next ten years. Indeed by 2015, it may seem inconceivable to people working in this area that something like the 'pill scare' actually happened.

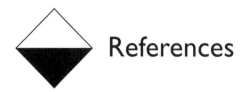

References

Abraham, C. and Sheeran, P. (1997) Cognitive representations and preventive health behaviour: a review, in K.J. Petrie and J. Weinman (eds) *Perceptions of Health and Illness: Current Research and Applications.* Amsterdam: Harwood Academic Publishers.

Abramsky, L. and Fletcher, O. (2002) Interpreting information: what is said, what is heard – a questionnaire study of health professionals and members of the public, *Prenatal Diagnosis,* 22: 1188–94.

Adams, J. (1995) *Risk.* London: Routledge.

Adams, J. (1998) A 'Richter scale for risk'? Scientific management of uncertainty versus management of scientific uncertainty, *Interdisciplinary Science Reviews,* 23: 146–55.

Akram, G. (2000) Over the counter medication: an emerging and neglected drug abuse, *Journal of Substance Use,* 5: 136–42.

Alaszewski, A. and Horlick-Jones, T. (2003) How can doctors communicate information about risk more effectively, *British Medical Journal,* 327: 728–31.

Albert, T. and Chedwick, S. (1992) How readable are practice leaflets? *British Medical Journal,* 305: 1266–8.

Alhakami, A.S. and Slovic, P. (1994) A psychological study of the inverse relationship between perceived risk and perceived benefit, *Risk Analysis,* 14: 1085–96.

Altmann, D.G., Schultz, K.F. and Moher, D. (2001) The revised CONSORT statement for reporting randomised trials, *Annals of Internal Medicine,* 134: 663–94.

Amery, W.K. (1999) Coming full circle in pharmacovigilance: communicating safety information to patients through patient package inserts, *Pharmacoepidemiology and Drug Safety,* 8: 121–9.

Arkes, H.R. and Blumer, C. (1985) The psychology of sunk cost, *Organizational Behaviour and Decision Processes,* 35: 124–40.

Armitage, C.J. and Conner, M. (2000) Attitudinal ambivalence: a test of three key hypotheses, *Personality and Social Psychology Bulletin,* 26: 1421–32.

Armstrong, K., Schwartz, J.S., Fitzgerald, G., Putt, M. and Ubel, P.A. (2002) Effect of framing as gain versus loss on understanding and hypothetical treatment choices: survival and mortality curves, *Medical Decision Making,* 22: 76–83.

Azjen, I. (1985) From intentions to action: a theory of planned behaviour, in J. Kuhl and J. Beckman (eds) *Action Control: From Cognitions to Behaviors*. New York: Springer Verlag.

Azjen, I. (1988) *Attitudes, Personality and Behaviour*. Milton Keynes: Open University Press.

Azjen, I. and Fishbein, M. (1970) Attitudes-behaviour relations: a theoretical analysis and review of empirical research, *Psychological Bulletin*, 84: 888–918.

Azjen, I. and Madden, T.J. (1986) Prediction of goal directed behaviour: attitudes, intentions and perceived behavioural control, *Journal of European Social Psychology*, 22: 453–74.

Barclay, P., Costigan, S. and Davies, M. (1998) Risk language and dialects: Lottery can be used to show risks, *British Medical Journal*, 316: 1243.

Barnes, J., Mills, S.Y., Abbott, N.C., Willoughby, M. and Ernst, E. (1998) Different standards for reporting ADRs to herbal remedies and conventional OTC medicines: face to face interviews with 515 users of herbal remedies, *British Journal of Clinical Pharmacology*, 45: 496–500.

Barnes, M.D., Penrod, C., Neiger, B.L., Merrill, R.M., Thackeray, R., Eggett, D.L. and Thomas, E. (2003) Measuring the relevance of evaluation criteria among health information seekers on the internet, *Journal of Health Psychology*, 8: 71–82.

Baron, J. (1994) Nonconsequentialist decisions, *Behavioral and Brain Sciences*, 17: 1–42.

Barratt, B., Kiefer, D. and Rabago, D. (1999) Assessing the risks and benefits of herbal medicine: an overview of the scientific evidence, *Alternative Therapies*, 5: 40–9.

Beardon, P.H., McGilchrist, M.M., McKendrick, A.D., McDevitt, D.G. and MacDonald, T.M. (1993) Primary non-compliance with prescribed medicines in primary care, *British Medical Journal*, 307: 846–8.

Beck, U. (1992) *Risk Society: Towards a New Modernity*. London: Sage.

Becker, G.S. (1976) *The Economic Approach to Human Behaviour*. Chicago, IL: University of Chicago Press.

Becker, M.H. and Rosenstock, I.M. (1984) Compliance with medical advice, in A. Steptoe and A. Mathews (eds) *Healthcare and Human Behaviour*. London: Academic Press.

Beckman, H.B. and Frankel, R.M. (1984) The effect of physician behaviour on the collection of data, *Annals of Internal Medicine*, 101: 692–6.

Begg, C., Cho, M. and Eastwood, S. (1996) Improving the quality of reporting of randomised control trials: the CONSORT statement, *Journal of the American Medical Association*, 276: 637–9.

Bennett, P. (1998) *Communicating about Risks to Public Health: Pointers to Good Practice*. London: Department of Health.

Bennett, P. and Calman, K. (1999) *Risk Communication and Public Health*. Oxford: Oxford University Press.

Bennett, P. and Murphy, S. (1997) *Psychology and Health Promotion*. Buckingham: Open University Press.

Bennett, P., Coles, D. and McDonald, A. (1999) Risk communication as a decision process, in P. Bennett and K. Calman (eds) *Risk Communication and Public Health*. Oxford: Oxford University Press.

Bental, D.S., Cawsey, A. and Jones, B. (1999) Patient information systems that tailor to the individual, *Patient Education and Counselling*, 36: 171–90.

Bergus, G.R., Levin, I.P. and Elstein, A.S. (2002) Presenting risks and benefits to patients – the effect of information order on decision making, *Journal of General Internal Medicine*, 17: 612–17.

Berland, G., Elliott, M., Algazy, J., Kravitz, R. *et al.* (2001) Health information on the internet: accessibility, quality and readability in English and Spanish, *Journal of the American Medical Association*, 285: 2612–21.

Bernardini, C., Ambrogi, V., Perioli, L., Tiralti, M.C. and Fardella, G. (2000) Comprehensibility of the package leaflets of all medicinal products for human use: a questionnaire survey about the use of symbols and pictograms, *Pharmacological Research*, 41: 679–88.

Berry, D.C. (in press) Interpreting information about medication side-effects: differences in risk perception and intention to comply when medicines are prescribed for adults or young children, *Psychology, Health and Medicine*.

Berry, D.C., Gillie, T. and Banbury, S.P. (1995) What do patients want to know about their medicines? An empirical study, *Expert Systems with Applications*, 8: 419–28.

Berry, D.C., Michas, I.C., Gillie, T. and Forster, M. (1997) What do patients want to know about their medicines and what do doctors want to tell them? A comparative study, *Psychology and Health*, 12: 467–80.

Berry, D.C., Michas, I.C. and DeRosis, F. (1998) Evaluating explanations about drug prescriptions: effects of varying the nature of information about side-effects and its relative position in explanations, *Psychology and Health*, 13: 767–84.

Berry D.C., Knapp, P.R. and Raynor, D.K. (2001) Is 15% very common: informing people about the risks of medication side-effects, *International Journal of Pharmacy Practice*, 10: 145–51.

Berry, D.C., Knapp, P. and Raynor, D.K. (2002a) Provision of information about drug side-effects to patients, *The Lancet*, 359: 853–4.

Berry, D.C., Raynor, D.K., Knapp, P.R. and Bersellini, E. (2002c) Official warnings on thromboembolism risk with oral contraceptives fail to inform users adequately, *Contraception*, 66: 305–7.

Berry, D.C., Michas, I.C. and Bersellini, E. (2003) Communicating information about medicine: the benefits of making it personal, *Psychology and Health*, 18: 127–39.

Berry, D.C., Raynor, D.K, Knapp, P.R. and Bersellini, E. (2003c) Patient understanding of risk: impact of EU guidelines and other risk scales for consumer medicines information, *Drug Safety*, 26: 1–11.

Berry, D.C., Holden, W. and Bersellini, E. (in press) Interpretation of recommended risk terms: differences between doctors and lay people, *International Journal of Pharmacy Practice*.

Bersellini, E. and Berry, D.C. (2004) Communicating information about medicines: the benefits of a benefit statement. Proceedings of the British Psychological Society 12: 35.

Bier, V.M. (2001) On the state of the art: risk communication to the public, *Reliability Engineering and System Safety*, 71: 139–50.

Bishop, P., Kirwan, J. and Windsor, K. (1996) *The ARC Patient Literature Evaluation Project*. Chesterfield: The Arthritis and Rheumatism Council.

Bissell, P., Ward, P.R. and Noyce, P.R. (2000) Mapping the contours of risk: consumer perceptions of non-prescription medicines, *Journal of Social and Administrative Pharmacy*, 17: 136–42.

Bjerrum, L. and Fogel, A. (2003) Patient information leaflets – helpful guidance or a source of confusion? *Pharmacoepidemiology and Drug Safety*, 12: 55–9.

Blanchard, C.G., Librecque, M.S., Ruckdeschel, J.C. and Blanchard, E.B. (1988) Information about decision-making preferences of hospitalized cancer patients, *Social Science and Medicine*, 27: 1139–48.

Blenkinsopp, A. and Bradley, C. (1996) Over the counter drugs: patients, society and the increase in self medication, *British Medical Journal*, 312: 629–32.

Bogardus, S.T. Jr., Holmboe, E. and Jekel, J.F. (1999) Perils, pitfalls, and possibilities in talking about medical risk, *Journal of the American Medical Association*, 281: 1037–41.

Bornstein, B.H. and Chapman, G.B. (1995) Learning lessons from sunk costs, *Journal of Experimental Psychology: Applied*, 1: 251–60.

Boyle, J. (1983) *Patient Information and Prescription Drugs: Parallel Surveys of Physicians and Pharmacists*. New York: Louis Harris & Associates.

Braddock, C.H., Edwards, K.A., Hasenberg, N.M., Laidley, T.L. and Levinson, W. (1999) Informed decision making in outpatient practice, *Journal of the American Medical Association*, 282: 2313–20.

Brase, G.L. (2002) Which statistical formats facilitate what decisions? The perception and influence of different statistical information formats, *Journal of Behavioral Decision Making*, 15: 381–401.

Breakwell, G.M. (1997) Frameworks for risk communication (introduction to symposium), *Risk Decision and Policy*, 2: 111–12.

British Medical Association (1990) *The BMA Guide to Living with Risk*. London: Penguin.

Britten, N., Stevenson, F.A., Barry, C.A., Barber, N. and Bradley, C.P. (2000) Misunderstandings in prescribing decisions in general practice: qualitative study, *British Medical Journal*, 320: 484–8.

Broemer, P. (2002) Relative effectiveness of differently framed health messages: the influence of ambivalence, *European Journal of Social Psychology*, 32: 685–703.

Bryant, G.D. and Norman, G.R. (1980) Expressions of probability: words and numbers, *New England Journal of Medicine*, 302: 411.

Buchanan, B., Moore, J., Forsythe, D., Carenini, G., Ohlsson, S. and Banks, G. (1995) An intelligent interactive system for delivering individualised information to patients, *Artificial Intelligence in Medicine*, 7: 117–54.

Burger, J.M. and Burns, L. (1988) The illusion of unique invulnerability and the use of effective contraception, *Personality and Social Psychology Bulletin*, 14: 264–70.

Busson, M. and Dunn, A.P. (1986) Patients' knowledge about prescribed medicines, *The Pharmaceutical Journal*, 17 May: 624–6.

Bynner, J. and Parsons, S. (1997) *It Doesn't Get Any Better: The Impact of Poor Basic Skills on the Lives of 37 Year Olds*. London: The Basic Skills Agency.

Calman, K.C. (1996) Cancer: science and society and the communication of risk, *British Medical Journal*, 313: 799–802.

Calman, K.C. (1998) *The Potential for Health: How to Improve the Nation's Health*. Oxford: Oxford University Press.

Calman, K.C. (2001) The William Pickles lecture-issues of risk: 'this unique opportunity', *British Journal of General Practice*, 51: 47–51.

Calman, K.C. (2002) Communication of risk: choice, consent and trust, *The Lancet*, 360: 166–8.

Calman K.C. and Royston, G.H. (1997) Risk language and dialects, *British Medical Journal*, 315: 939–42.

Calman, K.C. and Smith, D. (2001) Works in theory but not in practice? The role of the precautionary principle in public health policy, *Public Administration*, 79: 185–204.

Calman, K.C., Bennett, P.G. and Coles, D.G. (1999) Risk to health: some key issues in management, regulation and communication, *Health, Risk & Society*, 1: 107–16.

Campbell, M.K., DeVellis, B.M. and Stretcher, V.J. (1994) Improving dietary behaviour: effects of tailored messages in primary care, *American Journal of Public Health*, 84: 783–7.

Cameron, L.D. and Leventhal, H. (1995) Vulnerability beliefs, symptom experiences and the processing of threat information: a self-regulatory perspective, *Journal of Applied Social Psychology*, 25: 1859–83.

Cartwright, A. (1990) Medicine taking by people aged 65 or more, *British Medical Bulletin*, 46: 63–76.

Cassell, M.M., Jackson, C. and Cheuvront, B. (1998) Health communication on the internet: an effective channel for health behaviour change? *Journal of Health Communication*, 3: 71–9.

Cawsey, A., Jones, R.B. and McRoy, J. (2000) The evaluation of a personalised health information system for patients with cancer, *User Modeling and User Adapted Interaction*, 10: 47–72.

Centre for Health Quality Improvement (1997) *High Quality Matters* (newsletter Issue 1). Winchester: Centre for Health Quality Improvement.

Charles, C., Gafni, A. and Whelan, T. (1997) Shared decision-making in the medical encounter: what does it mean? (or it takes at least two to tango), *Social Science and Medicine*, 44: 681–92.

Charles, C., Whelan, T. and Gafni, A. (1999) What do we mean by partnership in making decisions about treatment? *British Medical Journal*, 319: 780–2.

Clark, D., Layton, D. and Shakir, S. (2001) Monitoring the safety of over the counter drugs, *British Medical Journal*, 323: 706–7.

Cleveland, W.S. and McGill, R. (1984) Graphical perception – the visual decoding of quantitative information on graphical displays of data, *Journal of the Royal Statistical Society, Series A: Statistics in Society*, 150: 192–229.

Cosmides, L. and Tooby, J. (1996) Are humans good intuitive statisticians after all? Rethinking some conclusions from the literature on judgement under uncertainty, *Cognition*, 58: 1–7.

Coulter, A. (1999) Paternalism or partnership? Patients have grown up – and there's no going back, *British Medical Journal*, 19: 719–20.

Coulter, A., Entwistle, V. and Gilbert, D. (1998) *Informing Patients: An Assessment of the Quality of Patient Information Materials*. London: King's Fund.

Covello, V.T. (1991) Risk comparisons and risk communication: issues and problems in comparing health and environmental risks, in R.E. Kasperson and P.J. Stallen (eds) *Communicating Risks to the Public: International Perspectives*, pp. 79–124. Dordrecht: Kluwer Academic Publishers.

Daltroy, L.H. (1993) Doctor–patient communication in rheumatological disorders, *Ballire's Clinical Rheumatology*, 7: 221–30.

Dantas, F. and Rampes, H. (2000) Do homeopathic medicines provoke adverse effects? A systematic review, *British Homeopathic Journal*, 89: S35–8.

Davison, C., Davey-Smith, G.D. and Frankel, S. (1991) Lay epidemiology and the prevention paradox – the implications of coronary candidacy for health education, *Sociology of Health and Illness*, 13: 1–19.

De Steno, D., Petty, R.E., Wegener, D.T. and Rucker, D.D. (2000) Beyond valence in the perception of likelihood: the role of emotion specificity, *Journal of Personality and Social Psychology*, 78: 397–416.

Dekker, F.W., Kaptein, A.A., van der Waart, M.A. and Gill, K. (1992) Quality of self care of patients with asthma, *Journal of Asthma*, 29: 203–8.

Department of Health (1992) *The Health of the Nation: A Summary of the Government's Proposals*. London: HMSO.

Department of Health (1998) *Our Healthier Nation*. London: HMSO.

Department of Health (2000) *National Plan for the NHS*. London: Department of Health.

Dickinson, D., Raynor, D.K. and Duman, M. (2001) Patient information leaflets for medicines: using consumer testing to determine the most effective design, *Patient Educational and Counselling*, 43: 147–59.

DiClemente, C.C. and Prochaska, J.O. (1982) Self change and therapy change of smoking behaviour: a comparison of change in cessation and maintenance, *Addictive Behaviours*, 7: 133–42.

Donovan, J.L. and Blake, D.R. (1992) Patient non-compliance: deviance or reasoned decision-making? *Social Science and Medicine*, 34: 507–13.

Douglas, M. (1992) *Risk and Blame: Essays in Cultural Theory*. London: Routledge.

Dowling, H. (1996) Consumer product information – where to from here? *Australian Journal of Hospital Pharmacy*, 26: 293–8.

Doyal, L. (2001) Informed consent: moral necessity or illusion? *Quality in Health Care*, 10: 29–33.

Doyle, J.K. (1997) Judging cumulative risk, *Journal of Applied Social Psychology*, 27: 500–24.

Eagley, A.H. and Chaiken, S. (1993) *The Psychology of Attitudes*. Forth Worth, TX: Harcourt Brace College Publishers.

Eddy, D.M. (1982) Probabilistic reasoning in clinical medicine, in D. Kahneman, P. Slovic and A. Tversky (eds) *Judgment Under Uncertainty: Heuristics and Biases*, pp. 249–68. Cambridge: Cambridge University Press.

Edelmann, R.J. (2000) *Psychosocial Aspects of the Health Care Process*. London: Prentice Hall.

Edwards, A. (2003) Communicating risks means that patients too have to live with uncertainty, *British Medical Journal*, 327: 691–2.

Edwards, A. and Bastian, H. (2001) Risk communication: making evidence part of patient choices, in A. Edwards and G. Elwyn (eds) *Evidence-based Patient Choice: Inevitable or Impossible?* pp. 144–60. Oxford: Oxford University Press.

Edwards, A. and Elwyn, G. (2001a) Understanding risk and lessons for clinical risk communication about treatment preferences, *Quality in Health Care*, 10, 9–13.

Edwards, A. and Elwyn, G. (2001b) Standardising risks: listen and don't mislead, *British Journal of General Practice*, 51: 259–60.

Edwards, A., Matthews, E., Pill, R. and Bloor, M. (1998a) Communication about risk: diversity among primary care professionals, *Family Practice*, 15: 296–300.

Edwards, A., Matthews, E., Pill, R. and Bloor, M. (1998b) Communication about risk: the responses of primary care professionals to standardizing the 'language of risk' and communication tools, *Family Practice*, 15: 301–7.

Edwards, A., Elwyn, G. and Stott, N. (1999) Communicating risk reductions: researchers should present results with both relative and absolute risks, *British Medical Journal*, 318: 603–4.

Edwards, A., Elwyn, G. and Stott, N. (2001) Researchers should present results with both relative and absolute risks, *British Medical Journal*, 318: 602.

Edwards, A., Elwyn, G. and Mulley, A. (2002) Explaining risks: turning numerical data into meaningful pictures, *British Medical Journal*, 324: 827–30.

Edwards, I.R. and Hugman, B. (1997) The challenge of effectively communicating risk-benefit information, *Drug Safety*, 17: 216–27.

Edwards, I.R., Wiholm, B.E. and Martinez, C. (1996) Concepts in risk-benefit assessment: a simple merit analysis of a medicine? *Drug Safety*, 15: 1–7.

Edwards, S., Lilford, R. and Hewison, J. (1998) The ethics of randomized control trials from the perspectives of patients, the public and healthcare professionals, *British Medical Journal*, 317: 1209–12.

Eisenberg, D.M., Davis, R.B. and Eltner, S.L. (1998) Trends in alternate medicine use in the US 1990–1997, *Journal of the American Medical Association*, 280: 1569–75.

Eiser, J.R., Eiser, C. and Pauwels, P. (1993) Skin cancer: assessing perceived and behavioural attitudes, *Psychology and Health*, 8: 393–404.

Ellen, S.P., Bone, P.F. and Stuart, E.W. (2001) How well do young people follow the label: an investigation of four classes of over the counter drugs, *Journal of Public Policy and Marketing*, 17: 70–85.

Elting, L.S., Martin, C.G., Cantor, S.B. and Rubenstein, E.B. (1999) Influence of data display formats on physician investigators' decisions to stop clinical trials: prospective trial with repeated measures, *British Medical Journal*, 318: 1527–31.

Emmons, K.M. (2000) Behavioural and social science contributions to the health of adults in the US, in B. Smedley and S.L. Syme (eds) *Promoting Health: Intervention Strategies from Social and Behavioural Research*, pp. 254–321. Washington, DC: National Academic Press.

Eng, T.R. (2001) *The eHealth Landscape: A Terrain Map of Emerging Health Information and Communication Technologies in Health and Healthcare*. Princeton, NJ: The Robert Wood Johnson Foundation.

Enlund, H., Vanio, K., Wallenius, S. and Poston, J.W. (1991) Adverse drug effects and the need for drug information, *Medical Care*, 29: 558–64.

Erev, I. and Cohen, B.L. (1990) Verbal and numerical probabilities: efficiency biases and the preference paradox, *Organizational Behaviour and Human Decision Processes*, 45: 1–18.

Ernst, D. (2002) Herbal medicine, *Complementary and Alternative Medicine*, 86: 149–61.

European Commission (1992) EEC Directive 92/27/EEC on labelling of medicinal products for human use and on package leaflets (OJ No. L113 of 30 April 1992).

European Commission (1998) A guideline on the readability of the label and package leaflet of medicinal products for human use. EC Pharmaceuticals Committee.

Eysenbach, G. (2000) Consumer health informatics, *British Medical Journal*, 320: 1713–16.

Fahey, T., Griffins, S. and Peters, T.J. (1995) Evidence based purchasing:

understanding results of clinical trials and systematic reviews, *British Medical Journal*, 311: 1056–9.

Fallowfield, L. (2001) Participation of patients in decisions about treatment for cancer (editorial), *British Medical Journal*, 323: 1144.

Finucane, M.L., Alhakami, A., Slovic, P. and Johnson, S.M. (2000) The affect heuristic in judgement of risks and benefits, *Journal of Behavioral Decision Making*, 13: 1–17.

Fischer, K. and Jungermann, H. (1996) Rarely occurring headaches and rarely occurring blindness: Is rarely=rarely? Meaning of verbal frequentistic labels in specific medical contexts, *Journal of Behavioral Decision Making*, 9: 153–72.

Fischoff, B. and MacGregor, D. (1983) Judged lethality: how much people seem to know depends upon how they are asked, *Risk Analysis*, 3: 229.

Fischoff, B., Bostrom, A. and Quadrel, M.J. (1993) Risk perception and communication, *Annual Review of Public Health*, 14: 183–203.

Fischoff, B., Slovic, P., Lichtenstein, S., Read, S. and Coombes, B. (1978) How safe is safe enough? A psychometric study of attitudes towards technological risks and benefits, *Policy Sciences*, 9: 127–52.

Floyd, D.L., Prentice-Dunn, S. and Rogers, R.W. (2000) A meta-analysis of research on protection motivation theory, *Journal of Applied Social Psychology*, 30: 407–29.

Flugstad, A.R. and Windschitl, P.D. (2003) The influence of reasons on interpretations of probability forecasts, *Journal of Behavioural Decision Making*, 16: 107–26.

Fontaine, K.R. and Smith, S. (1995) Optimistic bias in cancer risk perception: a cross national study, *Psychological Reports*, 77: 143–6.

Forrow, L., Taylor, W.C. and Arnold, R.M. (1992) Absolutely relative: how research results are summarised can affect treatment decisions, *The American Journal of Medicine*, 92: 121–4.

Fortin, J.M., Hirota, L.K., Bond, B.E., O'Connor, A.M. and Col, N.F. (2001) Identifying patient preferences for communicating risk estimates: a descriptive pilot study, *BMC Medical Information and Decision Making*, 1: 2.

Foucault, M. (1991) Governmentality, in G. Burchall, C. Gordon and P. Miller (eds) *The Foucault Effect: Studies in Governmentality*. Hemel Hempstead: Harvester Wheatsheaf.

Fox, C.R. and Irwin, J.R. (1998) The role of context in the communication of uncertain beliefs, *Basic and Applied Social Psychology*, 20: 57–70.

Fraenkel, L., Bogardus, S., Concato, J. and Felson, D. (2003) Risk communication in rheumatoid arthritis, *Journal of Rheumatology*, 30: 443–8.

French, J.F. and Adams, L.A. (2002) From analysis to synthesis: theories of health education, in D.F. Marks (ed.) *The Health Psychology Reader*. London: Sage.

Frewer, L.J. (1999) Public risk perception and risk communication, in P. Bennett and K. Calman (eds) *Risk Communication and Public Health*, pp. 20–32. Oxford: Oxford University Press.

Frewer, L.J. (2003) Trust, transparency and social context: implications for social amplification of risk, in N. Pidgeon, R.E. Kasperson and P. Slovic (eds) *The Social Amplification of Risk*. Cambridge: Cambridge University Press.

Fugh-Berman, A. (2000) Herb drug interactions, *The Lancet*, 355: 134–8.

George, L.F., Waters, W.E. and Nicholas, J.A. (1983) Prescription information leaflets, a pilot study in general practice, *British Medical Journal*, 287: 1193–6.

Giddens, A. (1990) *The Consequences of Modernity*. Cambridge: Polity Press.

Giddens, A. (1991) *Modernity and Self Identity*. Cambridge: Polity Press.

Gigerenzer, G. (2002) *Reckoning with Risk*. London: Penguin.

Gigerenzer, G. and Edwards, A. (2003) Simple tools for understanding risks: from innumeracy to insight, *British Medical Journal*, 327: 741–4.

Gigerenzer, G. and Goldstein, D.G. (1996) Reasoning the fast and frugal way: models of bounded rationality, *Psychological Review*, 103: 650–9.

Gilbertson, R.J., Harris, E., Pandey, S.K., Kelly, P. and Myers, W. (1996) Paracetamol use, availability and knowledge of toxicity among British and American adolescents, *Archives of Disease in Childhood*, 75: 194–8.

Gilovitch, T., Griffin, D. and Kahneman, D. (2002) *Heuristics and Biases: The Psychology of Intuitive Prediction*. Cambridge: Cambridge University Press.

Godin, G. and Kok, G. (1996) The theory of planned behavior: a review of its applications to health-related behaviors, *American Journal of Health Promotion*, 11: 87–98.

Gollwitzer, P.M. (1993) Goal achievement: the role of intentions, in W. Stroebe and M. Hewstone (eds) *European Review of Social Psychology*, 4: 141–85.

Gollwitzer, P.M. (1999) Implementation intentions: strong effects of simple plans, *American Psychologist*, 54: 493–503.

Green, E., Short, S.D., Duarte-Davidson, R. and Levy, L.S. (1999) Public and professional perceptions of environmental and health risks, in P. Bennett and K. Calman (eds) *Risk Communication and Public Health*. Oxford: Oxford University Press.

Gurm, H.S. and Litaker, D.G. (2000) Framing procedural risks to patients: is 99% safe the same as a risk of 1 in 100? *Academic Medicine*, 75: 840–2.

Gutteling, J.M. and Wiegman, O. (1996) *Exploring Risk Communication*. Dordrecht: Kluwer Academic Publishers.

Guttman, N. (2000) *Public Health Communication Intervention: Values and Dilemmas*. Thousand Oaks, CA: Sage.

Hall, A. (2001) The role of effective communication in obtaining informed consent, in L. Doyal and J.S. Tobias (eds) *Informed Consent in Medical Research*. London: BMJ Books.

Hall, J., Roter, D. and Katz, N. (1988) Meta-analysis of correlates of provider behaviour in medical encounters, *Medical Care*, 26: 657–75.

Halpern, D.F., Blackman, S. and Salzman, B. (1989) Using statistical risk information to assess oral-contraceptive safety, *Applied Cognitive Psychology*, 3: 251–60.

Hampson, S.E., Andrews, J.A., Lee, M.E., Foster, L.S., Glasgow, R.E. and Lichtenstein, E. (1998) Lay understanding of synergistic risk: the case of radon and cigarette smoking, *Risk Analysis*, 18, 343–50.

Hardey, M. (1999) Doctor in the house: the internet as a source of lay health knowledge and the challenge to expertise, *Sociology of Health and Illness*, 21: 820–35.

Harris, P. and Middleton, W. (1994) The illusion of control and optimism about health: on being less at risk but no more in control than others, *British Journal of Social Psychology*, 33: 369–86.

Harrison, J.A., Mullen, P.D. and Green, L.W. (1992) A meta-analysis of studies of the health belief model with adults, *Health Education Research*, 7: 107–16.

Hastie, R. (2001) Problems for judgement and decision making, *Annual Review of Psychology*, 52: 653–83.

Helweg-Larsen, M. and Shepperd, J.A. (2001) Do moderators of the optimistic bias affect personal or target risk estimates? A review of the literature, *Personality and Social Psychology Review*, 5: 74–95.

Hibbard, J.H., Slovic, P., Peters, E. and Finucane, M.L. (2002) Strategies for representing healthplan performance information to consumers: evidence from controlled studies, *Health Services Research*, 37: 291–313.

Hillman, M.J., Adams, J. and Whitelegg, J. (1990) *One False Move: A Study of Children's Independent Mobility*. London: Policy Studies Institute.

Hingorani, A.D. and Vallance, P. (1999) A simple computer program for guiding management of cardiovascular risk factors and prescribing, *British Medical Journal*, 318: 101–5.

Hinks, J.K., Eustace, J.K. and Wogalter, M.S. (1998) Do grables enable the extraction of quantitative information better than pure graphs or tables? *International Journal of Industrial Ergonomics*, 22: 439–47.

Hoffrage, U. and Gigerenzer, G. (1998) Using natural frequencies to improve diagnostic inferences, *Academic Medicine*, 73: 538–40.

Hoffrage, U., Lindsey, S., Hertwig, R. and Gigerenzer, G. (2000) Medicine: communicating statistical information, *Science*, 290: 2261–2.

Hollands, J.G. and Spence, I. (1998) Judging proportions from graphs: the summation model, *Applied Cognitive Psychology*, 12: 173–90.

Hoorens, V. and Buunk, B.P. (1993) Social comparisons of health risks: locus of control, the person-positivity bias and unrealistic optimism, *Journal of Applied Social Psychology*, 23: 291–302.

Horne, R. (1998) Adherence to medication: a review of existing research, in L.B. Myers and K. Midence (eds) *Adherence to Treatment in Medical Conditions*. Amsterdam: Harwood Academic Publishers.

Horne, R. and Weinman, J. (1998) Predicting treatment adherence: an overview of theoretical models, in L.B. Myers and K. Midence (eds) *Adherence to Treatment in Medical Conditions*. Amsterdam: Harwood Academic Publishers.

House of Lords (2000) *Complementary and Alternative Medicine*, Select Committee on Science and Technology, Sixth Report. London: HMSO.

Houts, P.S., Bachrach, R., Witmer, J.T., Tringali, C.A., Bucher, J.A. and Localio, R.A. (1998) Using pictographs to enhance recall of spoken medical instructions, *Patient Education and Counseling*, 35: 83–8.

Houts, P.S., Witmer, J.T., Egeth, H.E., Loscalzo, M.J. and Zabora, J.R. (2001) Using pictographs to enhance recall of spoken medical instructions II, *Patient Education and Counseling*, 43: 231–42.

Hughes, L., Whittlesea, C. and Luscombe, D. (2002) Patients' knowledge and perceptions of side effects of OTC medication, *Journal of Clinical Pharmacy and Therapeutics*, 27: 243–8.

Hupcey, J.E., Penrod, J., Morse, J.M. and Mitcham, C. (2001) An exploration and advancement of the concept of trust, *Journal of Advanced Nursing*, 36: 282–93.

Hux, J.E. and Naylor, C.D. (1995) Communicating the benefits of chronic preventive therapy: does the format of efficacy data determine patients' acceptance of treatment? *Medical Decision Making: An International Journal of the Society for Medical Decision Making*, 15: 152–7.

Inman, W.H. (1986) Risks in medical intervention: balancing therapeutic risks and benefits, in A. Worden (ed.) *The Future of Predictive Safety Evaluation*. Boston, MA: MTP Press.

International Medical Benefit Risk Foundation (1993) *Improving Patient Information and Education on Medicines.* Geneva: IMBRF.

Izzo, A.A. and Ernst, E. (2001) Interactions between herbal medicines and prescribed drugs: a systematic review, *Drugs*, 61: 2163–75.

Jadad, A.R. (1999) Promoting partnerships: challenges for the internet age, *British Medical Journal*, 319: 761–4.

Jadad, A.R. and Gagliardi, A. (1998) Rating health information on the internet: navigating to knowledge or to Babel? *Journal of the American Medical Association*, 279: 611–14.

Jungermann, H. (1997) When you can't do it right: ethical dilemmas of informing people about risk, *Risk Decision and Policy*, 2: 131–45.

Kahn, G. (1993) Computer based patient education: a progress report, *MD Computing*, 10: 93–100.

Kahneman, D. and Tversky, A. (1982) The psychology of preferences, *Scientific American*, 246: 160–7.

Kahneman, D. and Tversky, A. (1984) Choices, values, and frames, *American Psychologist*, 39: 341–50.

Kanvil, N. and Umeh, K.F. (2000) Lung cancer and cigarette use: cognitive factors, protection motivation and past behaviour, *British Journal of Health Psychology*, 5: 235–48.

Kaplan, R.M., Hammel, B. and Schimmel, L.E. (1985) Patient information processing and decision to accept treatment, *Journal of Social Behaviour and Personality*, 1: 113–20.

Kaplan, R.M., Sallis, J.F. and Patterson, T.L. (1993) *Health and Human Behaviour.* New York: McGraw-Hill.

Kasperson, R., Renn, O., Slovic, P., Brown, H., Emel, J., Goble, R., Kasperson, J. and Ratick, S. (1988) The social amplification of risk: a conceptual framework, *Risk Analysis*, 8: 177–87.

Kayne, S., Beattie, N. and Reeves, A. (1999) Survey of buyers of over the counter homeopathic medicines, *The Pharmaceutical Journal*, 263: 210–12.

Kenny, T., Wilson, R.G., Purves, I.N., Clark, J., Newton, L.D., Newton, D.P. and Moseley, D.V. (1998) A PIL for every ill? Patient information leaflets (PILs): a review of past, present and future use, *Family Practice*, 15: 471–9.

Kim, P., Eng, T.R., Deering, M.J. and Maxfield, A. (1999) Published criteria for evaluating health related web sites: review, *British Medical Journal*, 318: 647–9.

Kitching, J.B. (1990) Patient information leaflets: the state of the art, *Journal of the Royal Society of Medicine*, 83: 298–300.

Klein, C.T.F. and Helweg-Larsen, M. (2002) Perceived control and the optimistic bias: a meta-analytic review, *Psychology and Health*, 17: 437–46.

Klein, W.M. (1996) Maintaining self servicing social comparisons: biased reconstruction of one's past behaviours, *Personality and Social Psychology Bulletin*, 19: 732–9.

Knapp, P.R., Berry, D.C. and Raynor, D.K. (2001) Testing two methods of presenting side effect information about common medicines, *International Journal of Pharmacy Practice*, 9: R6.

Kong, A., Barnett, G.O., Mosteller, F. and Youtz, C. (1986) How medical professionals evaluate expressions of probability? *New England Journal of Medicine*, 315: 790–4.

Kosslyn, S.M. (1989) Understanding charts and graphs, *Applied Cognitive Psychology*, 3: 185–226.

Kreps, G.L. (2002) Consumer/provider communication research: a personal plea to address issues of ecological validity, relational development, message diversity and situational constraints, in D.F. Marks (ed.) *The Health Psychology Reader*. London: Sage Publications.

Kreps, G.L. (2003) The impact of communication on cancer risk incidence, morbidity, mortality, and quality of life, *Health Communication*, 15: 161–9.

Kreuter, M.W. and Holt, C.L. (2001) How do people process health information? Applications in an age of individualized communication, *Current Directions in Psychological Science*, 10: 206–9.

Kreuter, M.W., Strecher, V.J. and Glassman, B. (1999) One size does not fit all: the case for tailoring print materials, *Annals of Behavioral Medicine: A Publication of the Society of Behavioral Medicine*, 21: 276–83.

Lacy, C.R., Barone, J.A., Suh, D.C., Malini, P.L., Bueno, M. and Moylan, D.M. (2001) Impact of presentation of research results on the likelihood of prescribing medications to patients with left ventricular dysfunction, *American Journal of Cardiology*, 87: 203–7.

Lash, S. (1993) Reflexive modernisation: the aesthetic dimension, *Theory, Culture and Society*, 10: 1–23.

Lee, D.H. and Mehta, M.D. (2003) Evaluation of a visual risk communication tool: effects on knowledge and perception of blood transfusion risk, *Transfusion*, 43: 779–87.

Lek, Y. and Bishop, G.D. (1995) Perceived vulnerability to illness threats: the role of disease type, risk factor perception and attributes, *Psychological Health*, 10: 205–17.

Leung, W.C. (2002) Risk information study was marred by poor design, *British Journal of General Practice*, 51: 493–4.

Leventhal, H. (1993) Theories of compliance and turning necessities into preferences: applicaton to adolescent health action, in N.A. Krasnegor, L. Epstein, S.B. Johnson and S.F. Yaffe (eds) *Developmental Aspects of Health Behaviour*. New Jersey: Lawrence Erlbaum Associates.

Leventhal, H. and Cameron, L. (1987) Behavioral theories and the problem of compliance, *Patient Education and Counselling*, 10: 117–38.

Leventhal, H., Prohaska, T.R. and Hirschman, R.S. (1985) Preventative health behaviour across the life span, in J.C. Rosen and L.J. Solomon (eds) *Prevention in Health Psychology*. Hanover, NH: University Press of New England.

Leventhal, H., Benyamini, Y., Brownless, S. *et al.* (1997) Illness representations: theoretical foundations, in K.J. Petrie and J.A. Weinman (eds) *Perceptions of Health and Illness*, pp. 1–18. Amsterdam: Harwood.

Levin, P., Schneider, S.L. and Gaeth, G.J. (1998) All frames are not created equal: a typology and critical analysis of framing effects, *Organizational Behaviour and Human Decision Processing*, 76: 149–88.

Levy, J.A. and Strombeck, R. (2002) Health benefits and risks of the internet, *Journal of Medical Systems*, 26: 495–510.

Ley, P. (1973) Communication in the clinical setting, *British Journal of Orthodontics*, 1: 173–7.

Ley, P. (1988) *Communicating with Patients*. London: Croom Helm.

Ley, P. and Llewellyn, S. (1995) Improving patients' understanding, recall, satisfaction and compliance, in A. Broome and S. Llewellyn (eds) *Health Psychology: Process and Application*, 2nd edn. London: Chapman & Hall.

Lichtenstein, S., Slovic, P., Fischoff, B., Layman, M. and Combs, B. (1978) Judged frequency of lethal events, *Journal of Experimental Psychology: Human Learning and Memory*, 4: 551–78.

Linville, P., Fischer, G.W. and Fischoff, B. (1993) Perceived risk and decision making involving AIDS, in J.B. Pryor and G.D. Reeder (eds) *The Social Psychology of HIV Infection*. Hillsdale, NJ: Erlbaum.

Lipkus, I.M. and Hollands, J.G. (1999) The visual communication of risk, *Journal of National Cancer Institute Monographs*, 25: 149–62.

Lipkus, I.M., Samsa, G. and Rimer, B.K. (2001) General performance on a numeracy scale among highly educated samples, *Medical Decision Making*, 21: 37–44.

Livingstone, J., Axton, R.A., Mennie, M., Gilfallan, A. and Brock, D.J. (1993) A preliminary trial of couples screening for cystic fibrosis: designing an appropriate information leaflet, *Clinical Genetics*, 43: 57–62.

Lloyd, A., Hayes, P., Bell, P.R.F. and Naylor, A.R. (2001) The role of risk and benefit perception in informed consent for surgery, *Medical Decision Making*, 21: 141–9.

Lowenstein, G.F., Weber, E.U., Hsee, C.K. and Welch, N. (2001) Risk as feelings, *Psychological Bulletin*, 127: 267–86.

Lupton, D. (1999) *Risk*. London: Routledge.

Lyons, R.F., Rumore, M.M. and Merola, M.R. (1996) An analysis of drug information desired by the patient (are patients being told everything they wish to know under OBRA '90?), *Journal of Clinical Pharmacy and Therapeutics*, 21: 221–8.

MacFarlane, J.T., Holmes, W.F. and MacFarlane, R.M. (1997) Reducing reconsultations for acute lower respiratory tract illness with an information leaflet: a randomised controlled study of patients in primary care, *British Journal of General Practice*, 47: 719–22.

Maguire, P., Fairburn, S. and Fletcher, C. (1989) Consultation skills of young doctors: benefits of feedback training, in M. Stewart and D. Roter (eds) *Communicating with Patients*, pp. 124–37. London: Sage.

Maheswaren, D. and Meyers-Levy, L. (1990) The influence of message framing and issue involvement, *Journal of Marketing Research*, 27: 361–7.

Makoul, G., Arntson, P. and Schofield, T. (1995) Health promotion in primary care: physician-patient communication and decision making about prescription medications, *Social Science & Medicine*, 41: 1241–54.

Malenka, D.J., Baron, J.A., Johansen, S., Wahrenberger, J.W. and Ross, J.M. (1993) The framing effect of relative and absolute risk, *Journal of General Internal Medicine*, 8: 543–8.

Man-Song Hing, M., Laupacis, A., O'Connor, A., Biggs, J., Drake, E., Yetirsir, E. and Hart, R.G. (1999) A patient decision aid regarding antithrombotic therapy for stroke prevention in atrial fibrillation: a randomized control trial, *Journal of the American Medical Association*, 22: 737–43.

Marcus, B.H., Bock, B.C., Pinto, B.M. and Clark, M.W. (1996) Exercise initiation, adoption and maintenance, in J.L. van Raalte and B.W. Brewer (eds) *Exploring Sport and Exercise Psychology*, pp. 133–58. Washington, DC: American Psychological Association.

Markham, I.S. (1998) Ethical and legal issues, *British Medical Bulletin*, 54: 1011–21.

Markman, K.D., Gavinski, I., Sherman, S.J. and McMullen, M.N. (1995) The impact of perceived control on the imagination of better and worse possible worlds, *Personality and Social Psychology Bulletin*, 21: 588–95.

Marks, D.F., Murray, M., Evans, B. and Willig, C. (2000) *Health Psychology: Theory, Research and Practice*. London: Sage.

Marwick, C. (1997) MedGuide: at last a long sought opportunity for patient education about prescribed drugs, *Journal of the American Medical Association*, 277: 949–50.

Matarazzo, J.D. (1984) Behavioural health: a 1990 challenge for the health sciences professions, in J. Matarazzo, N.E. Miller, S.M. Weiss and J.A. Herd (eds) *Behavioural Health: A Handbook of Health Enhancement and Disease Prevention*, pp. 3–40. New York: John Wiley.

Mayberry, J.F. and Mayberry, M.K. (1996) Effective instructions for patients, *Journal of Royal College of Physicians*, 30: 205–8.

Mayer, J.D., Gaschke, Y.N., Braverman, D.L. and Evans, T.W. (1992) Mood congruent judgement is a general effect, *Journal of Personality and Social Psychology*, 63: 119–32.

Mazur, D.J. and Hickman, D.H. (1993) Patients' and physicians' interpretations of graphic data displays, *Medical Decision Making*, 13: 59–63.

Mazur, D.J. and Merz, J.F. (1994) Patients' interpretations of verbal expressions of probability: implications for securing informed consent to medical interventions, *Behavioral Science and Law*, 12: 417–26.

McCormick, J. (1996) Medical hubris and the public health: the ethical dimension, *Journal of Clinical Epidemiology*, 49: 619–21.

McElnay, J.C. and McCallion, R. (1998) Adherence and the elderly, in L.B. Myers and R. Midence (eds) *Adherence to Treatment in Medical Conditions*. London: Harwood.

McGinnis, J.M. and Foege, W.H. (1993) Actual causes of death in the US, *Journal of the American Medical Association*, 270: 2207–12.

McKechnie, S. and Davies, S. (1999) Consumers and risk, in P. Bennett and K.C. Calman (eds) *Risk Communication and Public Health*. Oxford: Oxford University Press.

McLeod, S. (1998) The quality of medical information on the internet: a new public health concern, *Archives of Opthalmology*, 116: 1663–5.

McNeil, B.J., Pauker, S.G., Sox, H.C. and Tversky, A. (1982) On the elicitation of preferences for alternative therapies, *New England Journal of Medicine*, 306: 1259–62.

McRoy, S., Liu-Perez, A. and Ali, S. (1998) Interactive computerised health care education, *Journal of the American Medical Informatics Association*, 5: 347–56.

Meara, J. (2002) Getting the message across: is communicating risk to the public worth it? *Journal of Radiological Protection*, 22: 79–85.

Medow, M.A., Wilt, T.J., Dysken, S., Hillson, S.D., Woods, S. and Borowsky, S.J. (2001) Effect of written and computerized decision support aids for the US Agency for Health Care Policy and Research depression guidelines on the evaluation of hypothetical clinical scenerios, *Medical Decision Making: An International Journal of the Society for Medical Decision Making*, 21: 344–56.

Mellors, B.A. (2000) Choice and the relative pleasure of consequences, *Psychological Bulletin*, 126: 910–24.

Meredith, P., Emberton, M., Wood, C. and Smith, J. (1995) Comparison of patients' needs for information on prostate surgery with printed materials provided by surgeons, *Quality in Health Care*, 4: 18–23.

Merz, J.F., Druzdel, M.J. and Mazur, D.J. (1991) Verbal expressions of probability in informed consent litigation, *Journal of Medical Decision Making*, 1: 273–81.

Meyer, J., Shinar, D. and Leiser, D. (1997) Multiple factors that determine performance with tables and graphs, *Human Factors*, 39: 268–86.

Miller, L.G., Liu, H., Hays, R.D., Golin, C.E., Zhishen, Y., Beck, K., Kaplan, A.H. and Wenger, N.S. (2003) Knowledge of antiretroviral regimen dosing and adherence: a longitudinal study, *Clinical Infectious Diseases*, 36: 514–18.

Milne, S., Sheeran, P. and Orbell, S. (2000) Prediction and intervention in health related behaviour: a meta-analytic review of protection motivation theory. *Journal of Applied Social Psychology*, 30: 106–43.

Misselbrook, D. (2001) *Thinking about Patients*. Newbury: Petroc Press.

Mohanna, K. and Chambers, R. (2001) *Risk Matters in Healthcare: Communicating, Explaining and Managing Risk*. Oxford: Radcliffe Medical Press.

Molenaar, S., Sprangers, M.A., Postma-Shuit, F.C., Rutgers, G.J., Noorlander, J., Hendriks, J. and De Haes, H.C. (2000) Feasibility and effectiveness of decision aids, *Medical Decision Making*, 20: 112–29.

Montgomery, A.A. and Fahey, T. (2001) How do patients' treatment preferences compare with those of physicians? *Quality in Health Care*, 10: 39–43.

Morgan, M.G. and Lave, L. (1990) Ethical considerations in risk communication practice and research, *Risk Analysis*, 10: 355–8.

Morris, L.A. (1989) Communicating adverse drug effects to patients, *Journal of Clinical Research and Drug Development*, 3: 53–65.

Morris, L.A. and Kanouse, D.E. (1982) Informing patients about drug side effects, *Journal of Behavioural Medicine*, 5: 363–73.

Mossman, J., Boudioni, M. and Slevin, M.L. (1999) Cancer information: a cost-effective intervention, *European Journal of Cancer*, 35: 1587–91.

Mottram, D.R. and Reed, C. (1997) Comparative evaluation of patient information leaflets by pharmacists, doctors and the general public, *Journal of Clinical Pharmacy Therapy*, 22: 127–34.

Moxey, L.M. and Sandford, A.J. (1993) Prior expectations and the interpretation of natural language quantifiers, *European Journal of Cognitive Psychology*, 5: 73–91.

Moxey, L.M. and Sandford, A.J. (2000) Communicating quantities: a review of psycholinguistic evidence of how expressions determine perspectives, *Applied Cognitive Psychology*, 14: 237–55.

Moynihan, R., Bero, L., Ross-Degnan, D., Henry, D., Lee, K., Watkins, J., Mah, C. and Soumerai, S. (2000) Coverage by the news media of the benefits and risks of medications, *New England Journal of Medicine*, 342: 1645–9.

Muhlhauser, I. and Berger, M. (2000) Evidence-based patient communication in diabetes, *Diabetes Medicine*, 17: 823–9.

Myers, L.B. (1995) Taking a healthy interest in psychology, *Pharmacy Journal*, 253: 783.

Myers, L.B. and Midence, K. (1998) Concepts and issues in adherence, in L.B. Myers and K. Midence (eds) *Adherence to Treatment in Medical Conditions*. Amsterdam: Harwood Academic Publishers.

Nakao, M.A. and Axelrod, S. (1983) Numbers are better than words: verbal specifications of frequency have no place in medicine, *American Journal of Medicine*, 74: 1061–5.

National Cancer Alliance (1996) *Patient Centred Cancer Services: What Patients Say*. Oxford: The National Cancer Alliance.

Natter, H.M. and Berry, D.C. (2004) Effects of baseline information when communicating risk reductions in the domain of health, *Proceedings of the British Psychological Society*, 12: 51.

Neuhauser, L. and Kreps, G.L. (2003) Rethinking communication in the e-health era, *Journal of Health Psychology*, 8: 7–23.

Newton, L., Newton, D., Clark, J., Kenny, T., Moseley, D., Purves, I. and Wilson, R. (1998) Patient information leaflets: producing understandable PILs, *Journal of Information Science*, 24: 167–81.

Nexoe, J., Gyrd-Hansen, D., Krapstrup, D., Krishiansen, I.S. and Nielson, J.B. (2002) Danish GP's perception of disease risk and benefit of prevention, *Family Practice*, 19: 3–6.

Noble, L.M. (1998) Doctor–patient communication and adherence to treatment, in L.B. Myers and K. Midence (eds) *Adherence to Treatment in Medical Conditions*. Amsterdam: Harwood Academic Publishers.

Nuovo, J., Melnikow, J. and Chang, D. (2002) Reporting number needed to treat and absolute risk reduction in randomised control trials, *Journal of the American Medical Association*, 287: 2813–15.

O'Connor, A.M. and Edwards, A. (2001) The role of decision aids in promoting evidence-based patient choice, in A. Edwards and G. Elwyn (eds) *Evidence-based Patient Choice: Inevitable or Impossible?* pp. 220–44. Oxford: Oxford University Press.

O'Connor, A.M., Rostom, A., Fiset, V., Tetroe, J., Entwistle, V., Llewellyn-Thomas, H., Holnes-Rovner, M., Barry, M. and Jones, J. (1999) Decision aids for patients facing health treatment or screening decisions: systematic review, *British Medical Journal*, 319: 731–4.

O'Connor, A.M., Legare, F. and Stacey, D. (2003) Risk communication in practice: the contribution of decision aids, *British Journal of Psychology*, 327: 736–40.

Ogden, J. (2000) *Health Psychology: A Textbook*, 2nd edn. Buckingham: Open University Press.

Ohnishi, M., Fukui, T., Matsui, K., Hira, K., Shinozuka, M., Ezaki, H. *et al.* (2002) Interpretation of and preference for probability expressions among Japanese patients and physicians, *Family Practice*, 19: 7–11.

Ong, L.M., de Haes, J.C., Hoos, A.M. and Lammes, F.B. (1995) Doctor–patient communication: a review of the literature, *Social Science and Medicine*, 40: 903–18.

PAGB (2001) *Annual Report, Proprietary Association of Great Britain*. London: PAGB.

Paling, J. (1997) *Up to Your Armpits in Alligators: How to Sort Out What Risks are Worth Worrying About*. Gainesville, FL: Risk Communication and Environmental Institute.

Paling, J. (2003) Strategies to help patients understand risks, *British Medical Journal*, 327: 745–8.

Pander Maat, H. and Klassan, R. (1994) Side effects of side effect information in drug information leaflets, *Journal of Technical Writing and Communication*, 24: 389–404.

Parducci, A. (1968) Often is often, *American Psychologist*, 24: 828.

Pates, R., McBride, A.J., Li, S. and Ramadan, R. (2002) Misuse of over the counter medicines: a survey of community pharmacies in a South Wales health authority, *The Pharmaceutical Journal*, 268: 179–82.

Payne, S. (2002) Balancing information needs: dilemmas in patient information leaflets, *Health Informatics Journal*, 8: 174–9.

Payne, S., Large, S., Jarrett, N. and Turner, P. (2000) Written information given to patients and families by palliative care units: a national survey, *The Lancet*, 355: 1792.

Pelham, B.W., Sumarta, T.T. and Myaskovsky, L. (1994) The easy path from many to much: the numerosity heuristic, *Cognitive Psychology*, 26: 103–33.

Peterson, C. and De Avila, M.E. (1995) Optimistic explanatory style and perception of health problems, *Journal of Clinical Psychology*, 51: 128–32.

Petrie, K.J. and Weinman, J. (eds) (1997) *Perceptions of Health and Illness: Current Research and Applications*. Amsterdam: Harwood Academic Publishers.

Petts, J. (1992) Incineration risk perceptions and public concern: experience in the UK improving risk communication, *Waste Management and Research*, 10: 169–82.

Pidgeon, N., Hood, C., Jones, D., Turner, B. and Gibson, R. (1992) Risk perception, in *Risk: Analysis, Perception and Management: A Report of the Royal Society Study Group*, pp. 89–134. London: Royal Society.

Pinn, G. (2001) Adverse effects associated with herbal medicine, *Australian Family Physician*, 30: 1020–5.

Pollard, P. and Evans, J. (1983) The role of 'representativeness' in statistical inference: a critical appraisal, in J. Evans (ed.) *Thinking and Reasoning*. London: Routledge.

Povey, R., Conner, M., Sparks, P., James, R. and Shepherd, R. (2000) Application of the theory of planned behaviour to two dietary behaviours: roles of perceived control and self-efficacy, *British Journal of Health Psychology*, 5: 121–39.

Putnam, S.M., Stiles, W.B., Jacob, C.M. and James, S.A. (1988) Teaching the medical interview: an intervention study, *Journal of General Internal Medicine*, 3: 38–47.

Quill, T.E. and Brody, H. (1996) Physician recommendations and patient autonomy: finding a balance between physician power and patient choice, *Annals of Internal Medicine*, 125: 763–9.

Quirt, C.F., Mackillop, W.J., Ginsburg, A.D., Sheldon, L., Brundage, M., Dixon, P. et al. (1997) Do doctors know when their patients don't? A survey of doctor–patient communication in lung cancer, *Lung Cancer*, 18: 1–20.

Raynor, D.K. (1992) Patient compliance: the pharmacist's role, *The International Journal of Pharmacy Practice*, 1: 126–35.

Raynor, D.K. (1998) The influence of written information on patient knowledge and adherence to treatment, in L.B. Myers and K. Midence (eds) *Adherence to Treatment in Medical Conditions*. Amsterdam: Harwood Academic Publishers.

Raynor, D.K. (2001) PILS – kill or cure? *Pharmacy Practice*, 2001: 116–18.

Raynor, D.K. and Knapp, P.R. (2000) Do patients see, read and retain new mandatory medicine information leaflets? *Pharmacy Journal*, 264: 268–70.

Reid, S. (2002) A survey of the use of over the counter medicines purchased in health stores in Central Manchester, *Homeopathics*, 91: 225–9.

Renn, O. and Levine, D. (1991) Credibility and trust in risk communication, in R.E. Kasperson and P.J.M. Stallen (eds) *Communicating Risks to the Public: International Perspectives*. Dordrecht: Kluwer.

Renooij, S. and Witteman, C. (1999) Talking probabilities: communicating probabilistic information with words and numbers, *International Journal of Approximate Reasoning*, 22: 169–94.

Richard, R. and Van der Pligt, J. (1991) Factors affecting condom use among adolescents, *Journal of Communication and Applied Social Psychology*, 1: 105–16.

Richards, T. (1990) Chasms in communication, *British Medical Journal*, 301: 1407–8.

Rimer, B. and Glassman, B. (1997) Tailored communication for cancer prevention in managed care settings, *Outlook*, 4: 5.

Ritov, I. and Baron, J. (1990) Reluctance to vaccinate: omission bias and ambiguity, *Journal of Behavioural Decision Making*, 3: 263–77.

Roberts, R., Towell, T. and Golding, J.F. (2001) *Foundations of Health Psychology*. Basingstoke: Palgrave.

Rogers, R.W. (1975) A protection motivation theory of fear appeals and attitude change, *Journal of Psychology*, 91: 93–114.

Rogers, R.W. (1983) Cognitive and physiological processes in fear appeals and attitude change: a revised theory of protection motivation, in J.R. Cacioppo and R.E. Petty (eds) *Social Psychology: A Source Book*. New York: Guilford Press.

Rose, G. (1985) Sick individuals and sick populations, *International Journal of Epidemiology*, 14: 32–8.

Rosenstock, I.M. (1966) Why people use health services, *Millbank Memorial Foundation Quarterly*, 44: 94–124.

Rosenstock, I.M. (1974) The health belief model and preventative health behaviour, *Health Education Monographs*, 2: 354–6.

Roter, D.L. and Hall, J.A. (1989) Studies of doctor–patients interaction, *Annual Review of Public Health*, 10: 163–80.

Roter, D.L. and Hall, J.A. (1992) *Doctors Talking with Patients/Patients Talking with Doctors*. Westport, CT: Auburn House.

Rothman, A.J. and Salovey, P. (1997) Shaping perceptions to motivate healthy behavior: the role of message framing, *Psychological Bulletin*, 121: 3–19.

Rothman, A.J. and Schwartz, N. (1998) Constructing perceptions of vulnerability: personal relevance and use of experiential information in health judgements, *Personality and Social Psychology Bulletin*, 24: 1053–64.

Rothman, A.J., Kelly, K.M., Weinstein, N.D. and O'Leary, A. (1999) Increasing the salience of risky sexual behaviour: promoting interest in HIV antibody testing among heterosexually active young adults, *Journal of Applied Social Psychology*, 29: 531–51.

Rottenstreich, Y. and Hsee, C.K. (2001) Money, kisses and electric shocks: on the affective psychology of risk, *Psychological Science*, 12: 185–90.

Rowe, G. and Wright, G. (2001) Differences in expert and lay judgements of risk: myth or reality? *Risk Analysis*, 21: 341–56.

Rutter, D. and Quine, L. (2002) *Changing Health Behaviour: Intervention and Research with Social Cognition Models*. Milton Keynes: Open University Press.

Sackett, D.L. and Haynes, R.B. (1976) *Compliance with Therapeutic Regimens*. Baltimore, MD: Johns Hopkins University Press.

Salovey, P., Rothman, A.J. and Rodin, J. (1998) Health behavior, in D.T. Gilbert, S.T. Fiske and L. Gardner (eds) *The Handbook of Social Psychology*, pp. 633–83. New York: Oxford University Press.

Salva, J.J. and Portell, F. (2001) *Homeopathics*. London: Cassell.

Sandman, P.M., Weinstein, N.D. and Miller, P. (1994) High-risk or low – how location on a risk ladder affects perceived risk. *Risk Analysis*, 14: 35–45.

Scharloo, M. and Kaptein, A. (1997) Measurement of illness perceptions in patients with chronic somatic illness: a review, in K.J. Petrie and J. Weinman (eds) *Perceptions of Health and Illness: Current Research and Applications*. Amsterdam: Harwood Academic Publishers.

Schechtman, E. (2002) Odds ratio, relative risk, absolute risk reduction and the use of number needed to treat – which of these should we use? *ISPOR Value in Health*, 5: 430–5.

Schneider, C.E. (1998) *The Practice of Autonomy: Patients, Doctors & Medical Decisions*. Oxford: Oxford University Press.

Schriver, K.A. (1997) *Dynamics in Document Design*. Chichester: John Wiley.

Schwartz, L.M., Woloshin, S., Black, W.C. and Welch, H.G. (1997) The role of numeracy in understanding the benefit of screening mammography, *Annals of Internal Medicine*, 127: 966–72.

Schwartz, N. and Vaughn, L.A. (2002) The availability heuristic revisited: ease of recall and content of recall as distinct sources of information, in T. Gilovitch, D. Griffin and D. Kahneman (eds) *Heuristics and Biases: The Psychology of Intuitive Judgement*. Cambridge: Cambridge University Press.

Schwarzer, R. (1992) Self-efficacy in the adoption and maintenance of health behaviours: theoretical approaches and a new model, in R. Schwarzer (ed.) *Self-efficacy: Thought Control of Action*. Washington, DC: Hemisphere.

Sellu, D.P. (1987) Computer generated information leaflets for surgical patients, *British Journal of Clinical Practice*, 41: 612–17.

Semple, C.J. and McGowan, B. (2002) Need for appropriate written information for patients with particular reference to head and neck cancer, *Journal of Clinical Nursing*, 11: 585–93.

Shaklee, H. and Fischhoff, B. (1990) The psychology of contraceptive surprises – cumulative risk and contraceptive effectiveness, *Journal of Applied Social Psychology*, 20: 385–403.

Sheen, C.L. and Colin-Jones, D.G. (2001) Over the counter drugs and the gastro-intestinal tract, *Alimentary Pharmacology and Therapy*, 15: 1263–70.

Sheeran, P. (2002) Intention-behavior relations: a conceptual and empirical review, in W. Stroebe and M. Hewstone (eds) *European Review of Social Psychology*, pp. 1–36. Chichester: Wiley.

Sheeran, P. and Abraham, C. (1996) The health belief model, in M. Conner and P. Norman (eds) *Predicting Health Behaviours*, pp. 23–61. Buckingham: Open University Press.

Sheeran, P. and Orbell, S. (2000) Self-schemas and the theory of planned behaviour, *European Journal of Social Psychology*, 30: 533–50.

Shepherd, R. (1999) Social determinants of food choice, *Proceedings of the Nutrition Society*, 58: 807–12.

Sheridan, S.L. and Pignone, M. (2002) Numeracy and the medical student's ability to Interpret data, *Effective Clinical Practice*, 5: 35–40.

Simpson, M., Buckman, R., Stewart, M., Maguire, P., Lipkin, M., Novack, D. and Till, J. (1991) Doctor–patient communication: the Toronto Consensus Statement, *British Medical Journal*, 303: 1385–7.

Sinclair, H.K., Bond, C.M. and Hannaford, P.C. (2000) NSAIDs: improving patient care, *The Pharmaceutical Journal*, 265: 718.

Sjoberg, L. (1997) Explaining risk perception: an empirical evaluation of cultural theory, *Risk, Decision and Policy*, 2: 113–30.

Skinner, C.S., Campbell, M.K., Rimer, B.K., Curry, S. and Prochaska, J.O. (1999) How effective is tailored print communication? *Annals of Behavioral Medicine*, 21: 290–8.

Skolbekken, J.A. (1995) The risk epidemic in medical journals, *Social Science and Medicine*, 40: 291–305.

Sleath, B., Rubin, R.H., Campbell, W., Gwyther, L. and Clark, T. (2001) Physician-patient communication about over the counter medicines, *Social Science and Medicine*, 53: 357–69.

Sless, D. (2001) Usable written information for patients, *Medical Journal of Australia*, 174: 557–8.

Sless, D. and Wiseman, R. (1994) *Writing about Medicines for People: Usability Guidelines and Glossary for Consumer Product Information*. Canada: AGPS.

Slovic, P. (1987) Perception of risk, *Science*, 236, 280–5.

Slovic, P. (2000) *The Perception of Risk*. London: Earthscan Publications.

Slovic, P., Fischoff, B. and Lichtenstein, S. (1980) *Expressed Preferences* (report number 80–1). Eugene, OR: Decision Research.

Slovic, P., Flynn, J. and Laynan, M. (1991a) Perceived risk, trust and the politics of nuclear waste, *Science*, 254: 1603–7.

Slovic, P., Kraus, N., Lappe, H. and Major, M. (1991b) Risk perception of prescription drugs: report on a survey in Canada, *Canadian Journal of Public Health*, 82: 515–20.

Spence, I. and Lewandowsky, S. (1991) Displaying proportions and percentages, *Applied Cognitive Psychology*, 5: 61–77.

Squier, R.W. (1990) A model of empathic understanding and adherence to treatment regimens in practitioner-patient relationships, *Social Science and Medicine*, 30: 325–39.

Stanley, M.A. and Maddux, J.E. (1986) Cognitive processes in health enhancement: investigating a combined protection motivation and self efficacy model, *Basic and Applied Social Psychology*, 7: 101–13.

Starr, C. (1969) Social benefit versus technological risk, *Science*, 165: 1232–8.

Stevenson, F.A., Barry, C.A., Britten, N., Barber, N. and Bradley, C.P. (2000) Doctor–patient communication about drugs: the evidence for shared decision making, *Social Science and Medicine*, 50: 829–40.

Stewart, M.A. (1995) Effective physician-patient communication and health outcomes: a review, *Canadian Medical Association Journal*, 152: 1423–33.

Stone, E.R., Yates, J.F. and Parker, A.M. (1997) Effects of numerical and graphical displays on professed risk-taking behavior, *Journal of Experimental Psychology: Applied*, 3: 243–56.

Straus, S.E. (2002) Individualizing treatment decisions – the likelihood of being helped or harmed, *Evaluation and The Health Professions*, 25: 210–24.

Stroebe, W. (2000) *Social Psychology and Health*, 2nd edn. Buckingham: Open University Press.

Strull, W.M., Lo, B. and Charles, G. (1984) Do patients want to participate in medical decision making? *Journal of the American Medical Association*, 252: 2990–4.

Sutherland, H.J., Llewellyn-Thomas, H.A., Lockwood, G.A., Tritchler, D.L. and Till, J.E. (1989) Cancer patients: their desire for information and participation in treatment decisions, *Journal of the Royal Society of Medicine*, 82: 260–3.

Sutton, S. (1998) Predicting and explaining intentions and behavior: how well are we doing? *Journal of Applied Social Psychology*, 28: 1317–38.

Sutton, S. (2000) A critical review of the transtheoretical model applied to smoking cessation, in P. Norman, C. Abraham and M. Conner (eds) *Understanding and Changing Health Behaviour: From Health Beliefs to Self-Regulation*. Amsterdam: Harwood.

Sutton, S. (2001) Back to the drawing board? A review of applications of the transtheoretical model to substance use, *Addiction*, 96: 175–86.

Sutton, S. (2002) Using social cognition models to develop health behaviours and interventions: problems and assumptions, in D. Rutter and L. Quine (eds) *Changing Health Behaviour: Intervention and Research with Social Cognition Models*. Buckingham: Open University Press.

Svarstad, B.L. (1976) Physician-patient conformity with medical advice, in D. Mechanic (ed.) *Growth of Bureaucratic Medicine*. New York: Wiley.

Tavana, M., Kennedy, D.T. and Mohebb, B. (1997) An applied study using the analytic hierarchy process to translate common verbal phrases to numerical probabilities, *Journal of Behavioural Decision Making*, 10: 133–50.

Thomas, K.J., Nicholl, J.P. and Coleman, P. (2001) Use and expenditure on complementary medicine in England: a population based survey, *Complementary Therapies in Medicine*, 9: 2–11.

Timmermans, D. (1994) The roles of experience and domain of expertise in using numerical and verbal probability terms in medical decisions, *Medical Decision Making*, 14: 146–56.

Tomassoni, A.J. and Simone, K. (2001) Herbal medicines for children: an illusion of safety? *Current Opinion in Pediatrics*, 13: 162–9.

Tones, K. (1998) Health promotion: empowering choice, in L.B. Myers and K. Midence (eds) *Adherence to Treatment in Medical Conditions*. Amsterdam: Harwood Academic Publishers.

Tones, K. and Tilford, S. (2001) *Health Promotion: Effectiveness, Efficiency and Equity*, 3rd edn. Cheltenham: Nelson Thornes.

Toogood, J.H. (1980) What do you mean by 'usually'? *The Lancet*, 1: 1094.

Traynor, K. (2002) Drug information leaflets for consumers need improvement, FDA says, *American Journal of Health Systems Pharmacy*, 59: 1498–501.

Triandis, H. (1980) Values, attitudes and interpersonal behaviour, in H. Howe and M. Page (eds) *Nebraska Symposium on Motivation*, pp. 195–259. Lincoln, NE: University of Nebraska Press.

Tversky, A. and Kahneman, D. (1974) Judgement under uncertainty: heuristics and biases, *Science*, 185: 1124–31.

Tyler, V.E. (2000) Herbal medicine: from the past to the future, *Public Health Nutrition*, 3: 447–52.

US Department of Health and Human Sciences (1996) Prescription drug information for patients: notice of request for collaboration to develop an action plan, *Federal Regulations*, 61: 43769–70.

Vander Stichele, R.H., Vandierendonck, A., DeVooght, G., Reynvoet, B. and Lammerlyn, J. (2002) Impact of benefit messages in patient package inserts on subjective drug perception, *Drug Information Journal*, 36: 201–8.

Veatch, R.M. (1993) Benefit/risk assessment: what patients can know that scientists cannot, *Drug Information Journal*, 27: 1021–9.

Verplanken, B. (1997) The effects of catastrophic potential on the interpretation of numerical probabilities of the occurrence of hazards. *Journal of Applied Social Psychology*, 27: 1453–67.

Vuckovic, N. and Nichter, M. (1997) Changing patterns of pharmaceutical practice in the United States, *Social Science and Medicine*, 44: 1285–302.

Wallsten, T.S. and Budescu, D.V. (1990) Quantifying probability expressions: a comment, *Statistical Science*, 5: 23–6.

Wallsten, T.S., Fillenbaum, S. and Cox, J.A. (1986) Base rate effects on the interpretations of probability and frequency expressions, *Journal of Memory and Language*, 25: 571–87.

Wallsten, T.S., Budescu, D.V., Zwick, R. and Kemp, S.M. (1993) Preferences and reasons for communicating probabilistic information in verbal or numerical terms, *Bulletin of the Psychonomic Society*, 31: 135–8.

Weber, E.U. and Hilton, D.J. (1990) Contextual effects in the interpretations of probability words – perceived base rate and severity of events, *Journal of Experimental Psychology: Human Perception and Performance*, 16: 781–9.

Weinstein, N.D. (1982) Unrealistic optimism and susceptibility to health problems, *Journal of Behavioural Medicine*, 5: 441–60.

Weinstein, N.D. (1987) Unrealistic optimism and susceptibility to health problems: conclusions from a community-wide sample, *Journal of Behavioural Medicine*, 10: 481–500.

Weinstein, N.D. (1988) The precaution adoption process, *Health Psychology*, 7: 355–86.

Weinstein, N.D. (1989) Optimistic biases about personal risks, *Science*, 246: 1232–3.

Weinstein, N.D. and Klein, W.M. (1995) Resistance of personal risk perceptions to debiasing interventions, *Health Psychology*, 14: 132–40.

Weinstein, N.D. and Lyon, J.E. (1999) Mindset, optimistic bias about personal risk and health protective behaviour, *British Journal of Health Psychology*, 4: 289–300.

Weinstein, N.D., Rothman, A.J. and Sutton, S.R. (1998) Stage theories of health behaviour: conceptual and methodological issues, *Health Psychology*, 17: 290–9.

Weinstein, N.D., Lyon, J.E., Rothman, A.J. and Cuite, C.L. (2000) Changes in perceived vulnerability following natural disasters, *Journal of Social and Clinical Psychology*, 19: 372–95.

Williams, S., Weinman, J. and Dale, J. (1998) Doctor–patient communication and patient satisfaction: a review, *Family Practice*, 15: 480–92.

Wilson, M., Robinson, E.J., Blenkinsopp, A. and Panton, R. (1992) Customers' recall of information given in community pharmacies, *International Journal of Pharmacy Practice*, 1: 52–9.

Windschitl, P.D. and Weber, E.U. (1999) The interpretation of 'likely' depends on the context, but 70% is 70% right? The influence of associative processes on perceived certainty, *Journal of Experimental Psychology: Learning, Memory and Cognition*, 25: 1514–33.

Windschitl, P.D. and Wells, G.L. (1996) Measuring psychological uncertainty: verbal versus numeric methods, *Journal of Experimental Psychology: Applied*, 2: 343–64.

Windschitl, P.D., Martin, R. and Flugstad, A.R. (2002) Context and the interpretation of likelihood information: the role of intergroup comparisons on perceived vulnerability, *Journal of Personality and Social Psychology*, 82: 742–55.

Woloshin, S., Schwartz, L.M., Byram, S., Fischoff, B. and Welch, H.G. (2000) A new scale for assessing perceptions of chance: a validation study, *Medical Decision Making*, 20: 298–307.

World Health Organization (1948) *Preamble of the Constitution of the World Health Organization.* Copenhagen: World Health Organization.

World Health Organization (1991) *Revised Targets for Health in all Europe.* Copenhagen: World Health Organization.

Wright, P. (1998) Designing healthcare advice for the public, in F. Durso (ed.) *Handbook of Applied Cognition.* Chichester: Wiley.

Wright, P., Jansen, C. and Wyatt, J.C. (1998) How to limit clinical errors in interpretation of data, *The Lancet,* 352: 1539–43.

Yamagishi, K. (1997) When a 12.86% mortality is more dangerous than 24.14%: Implications for risk communication, *Applied Cognitive Psychology,* 11: 495–506.

Ziegler, D.K., Moiser, M.C., Buenaver, M. and Okuyemi, K. (2001) How much information about adverse effects of medications do patients want from physicians? *Archives of Internal Medicine,* 161: 706–13.

Author index

Subject index

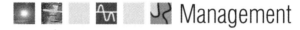
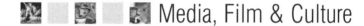
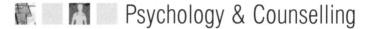
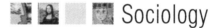
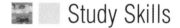
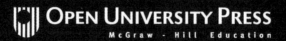
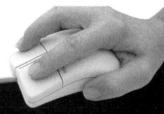